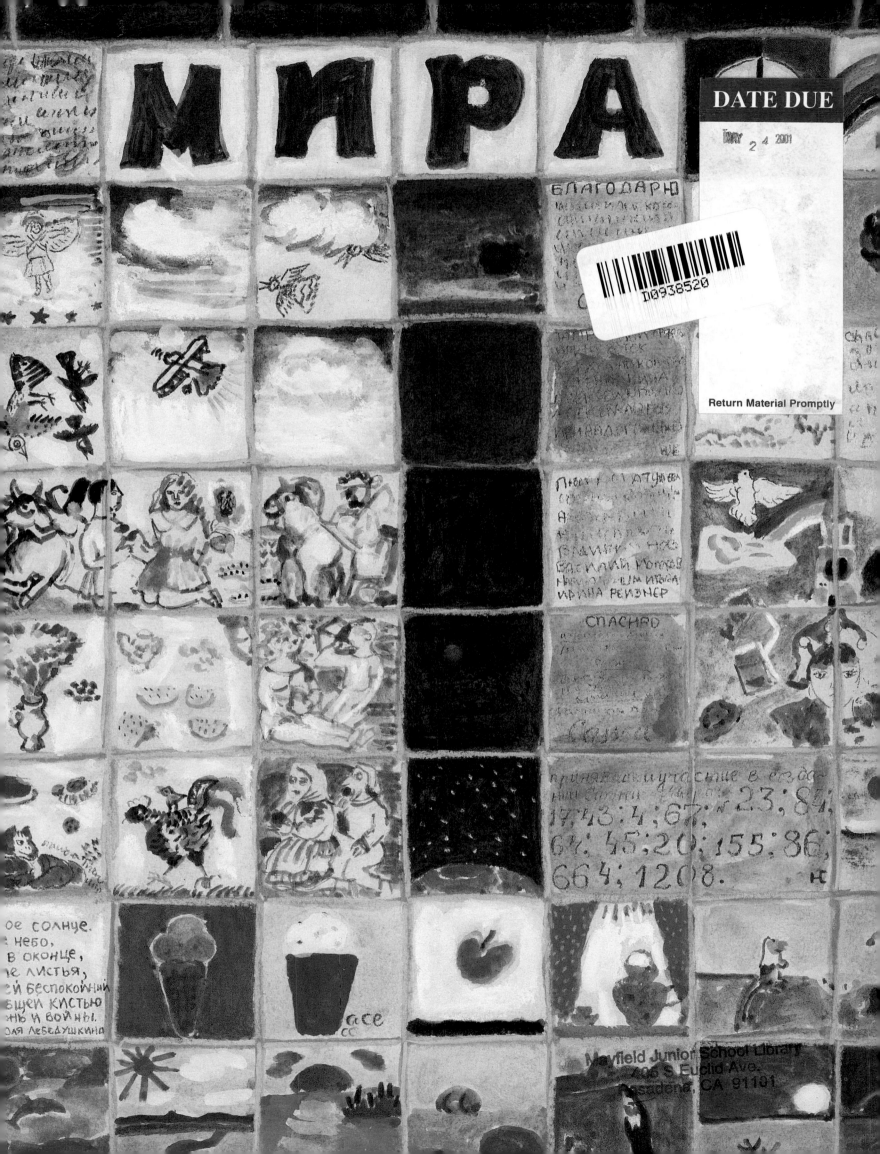

DATE DUE

MAY 2 4 2001

D0938520

Return Material Promptly

Mayfield Junior School Library
405 S. Euclid Ave.
Pasadena, CA 91101

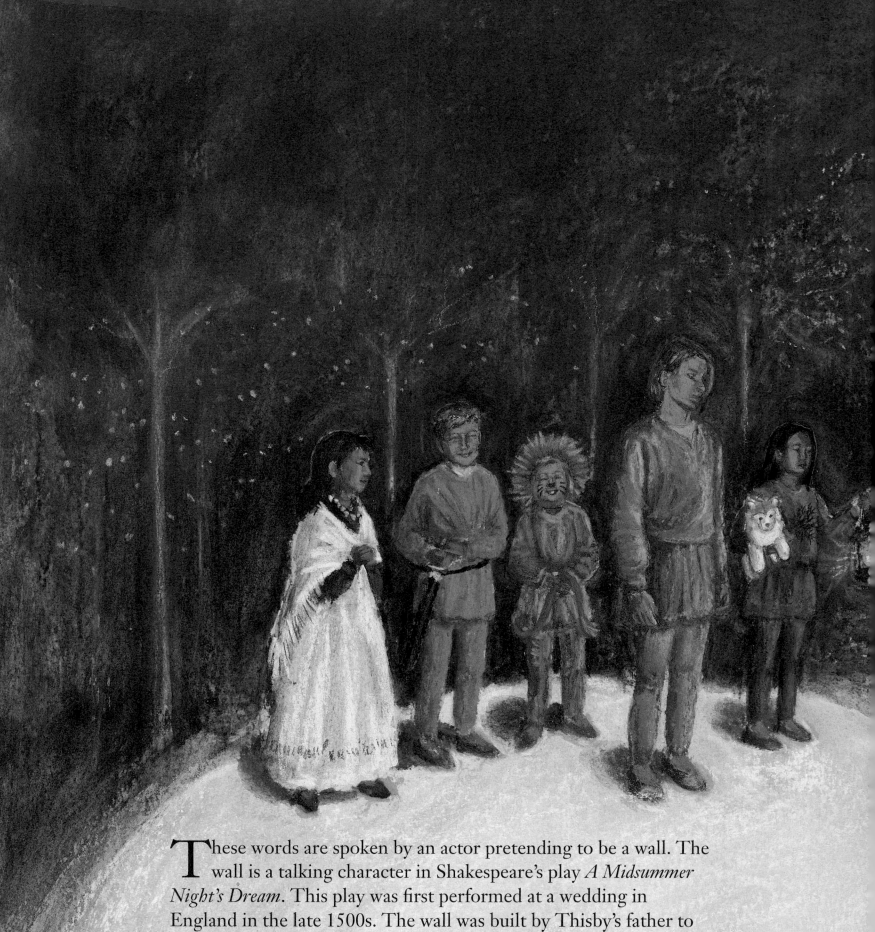

These words are spoken by an actor pretending to be a wall. The wall is a talking character in Shakespeare's play *A Midsummer Night's Dream*. This play was first performed at a wedding in England in the late 1500s. The wall was built by Thisby's father to try to prevent her from visiting Pyramus, her boyfriend.

The "talking wall" in Shakespeare's play tells a story. Many other walls all over the world also tell stories. Some of these stories are ancient and have been told for a long time, while other stories are newer and have just begun to be told.

Margy Burns Knight *Illustrated by* **Anne Sibley O'Brien**

Talking Walls
The Stories Continue

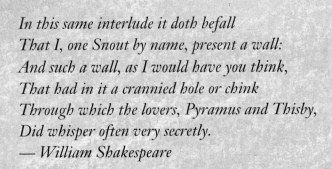

In this same interlude it doth befall
That I, one Snout by name, present a wall:
And such a wall, as I would have you think,
That had in it a crannied hole or chink
Through which the lovers, Pyramus and Thisby,
Did whisper often very secretly.
— William Shakespeare

Tilbury House, Publishers • Gardiner, Maine

Mayfield Junior School Library
405 S Euclid Ave.
Pasadena, CA 91101

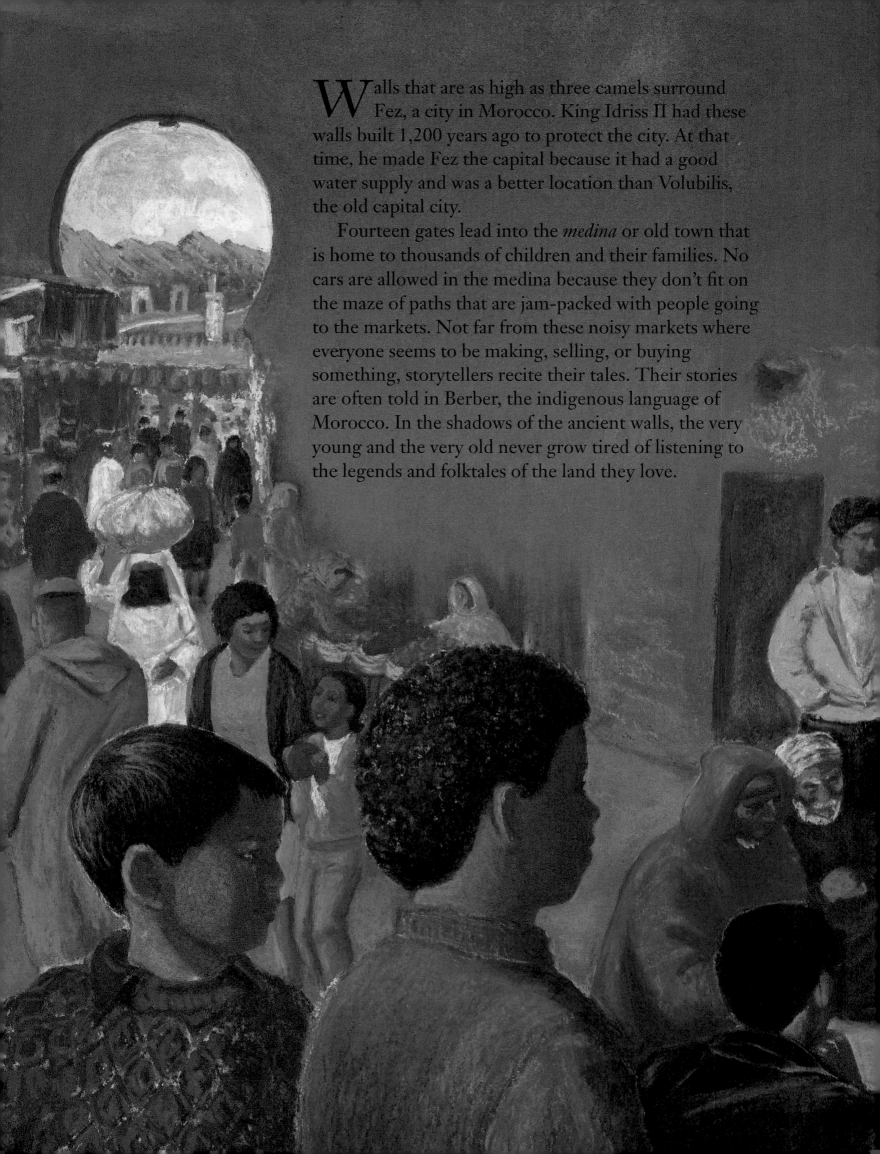

Walls that are as high as three camels surround Fez, a city in Morocco. King Idriss II had these walls built 1,200 years ago to protect the city. At that time, he made Fez the capital because it had a good water supply and was a better location than Volubilis, the old capital city.

Fourteen gates lead into the *medina* or old town that is home to thousands of children and their families. No cars are allowed in the medina because they don't fit on the maze of paths that are jam-packed with people going to the markets. Not far from these noisy markets where everyone seems to be making, selling, or buying something, storytellers recite their tales. Their stories are often told in Berber, the indigenous language of Morocco. In the shadows of the ancient walls, the very young and the very old never grow tired of listening to the legends and folktales of the land they love.

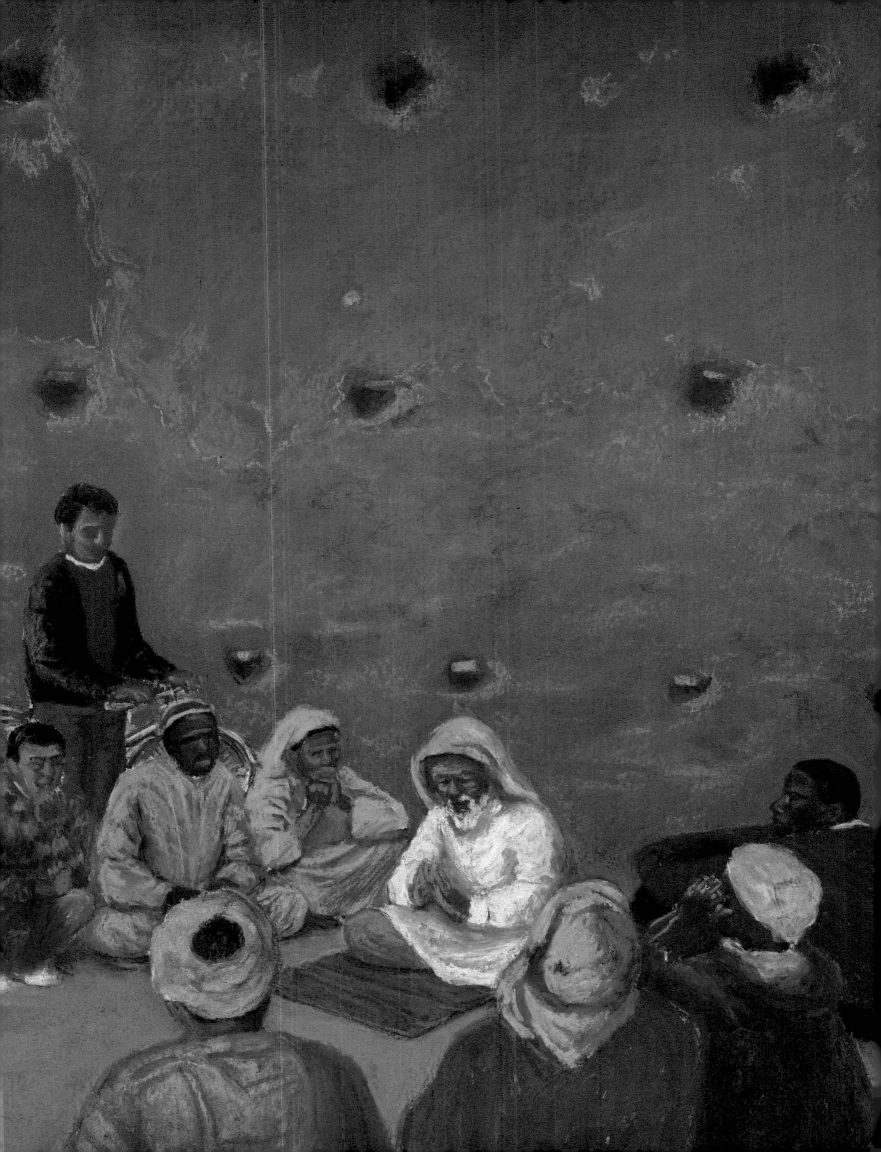

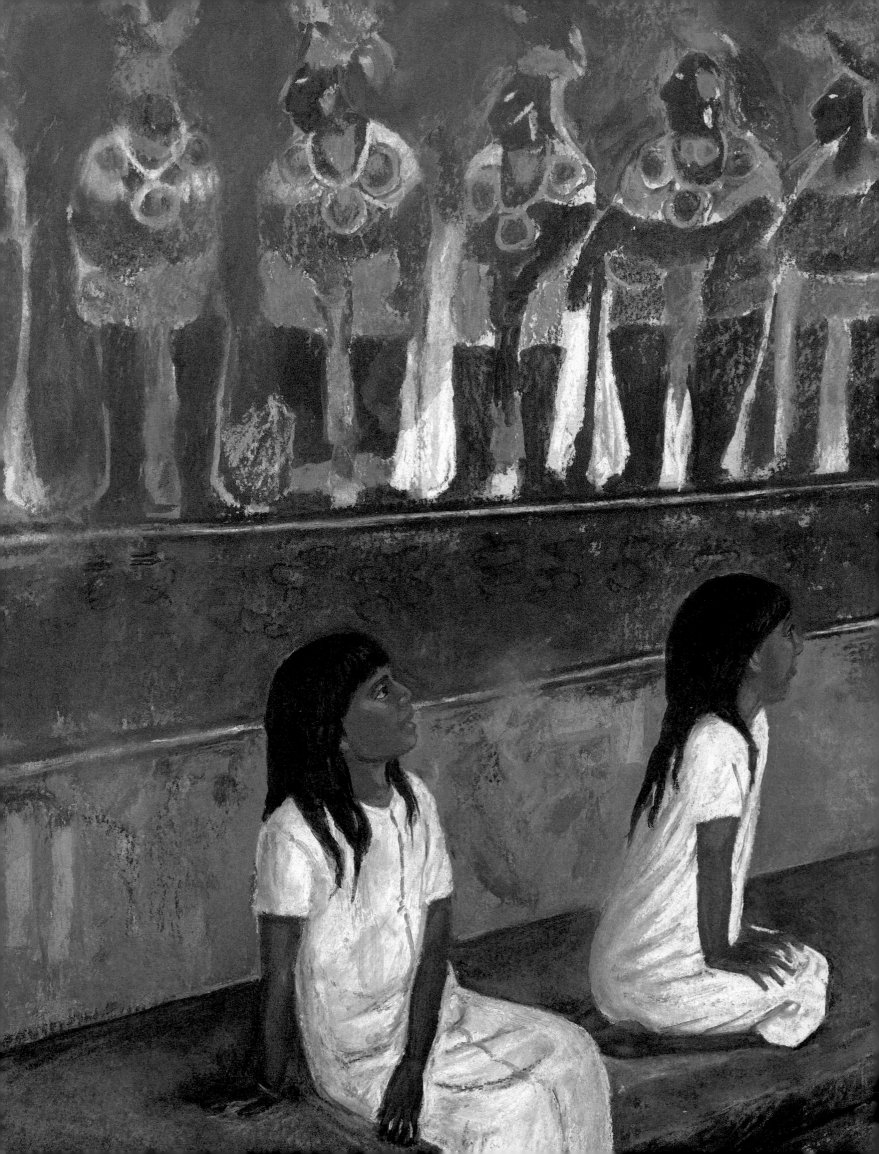

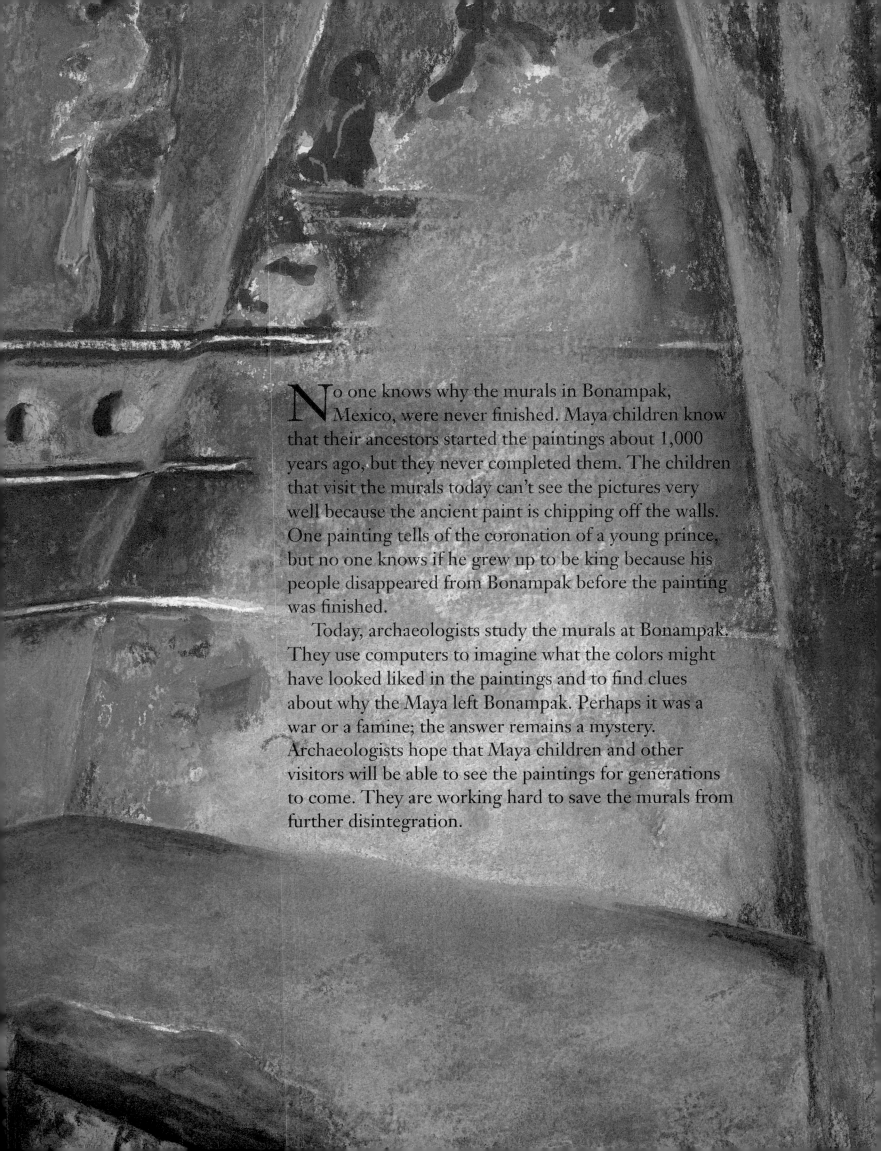

No one knows why the murals in Bonampak, Mexico, were never finished. Maya children know that their ancestors started the paintings about 1,000 years ago, but they never completed them. The children that visit the murals today can't see the pictures very well because the ancient paint is chipping off the walls. One painting tells of the coronation of a young prince, but no one knows if he grew up to be king because his people disappeared from Bonampak before the painting was finished.

Today, archaeologists study the murals at Bonampak. They use computers to imagine what the colors might have looked liked in the paintings and to find clues about why the Maya left Bonampak. Perhaps it was a war or a famine; the answer remains a mystery. Archaeologists hope that Maya children and other visitors will be able to see the paintings for generations to come. They are working hard to save the murals from further disintegration.

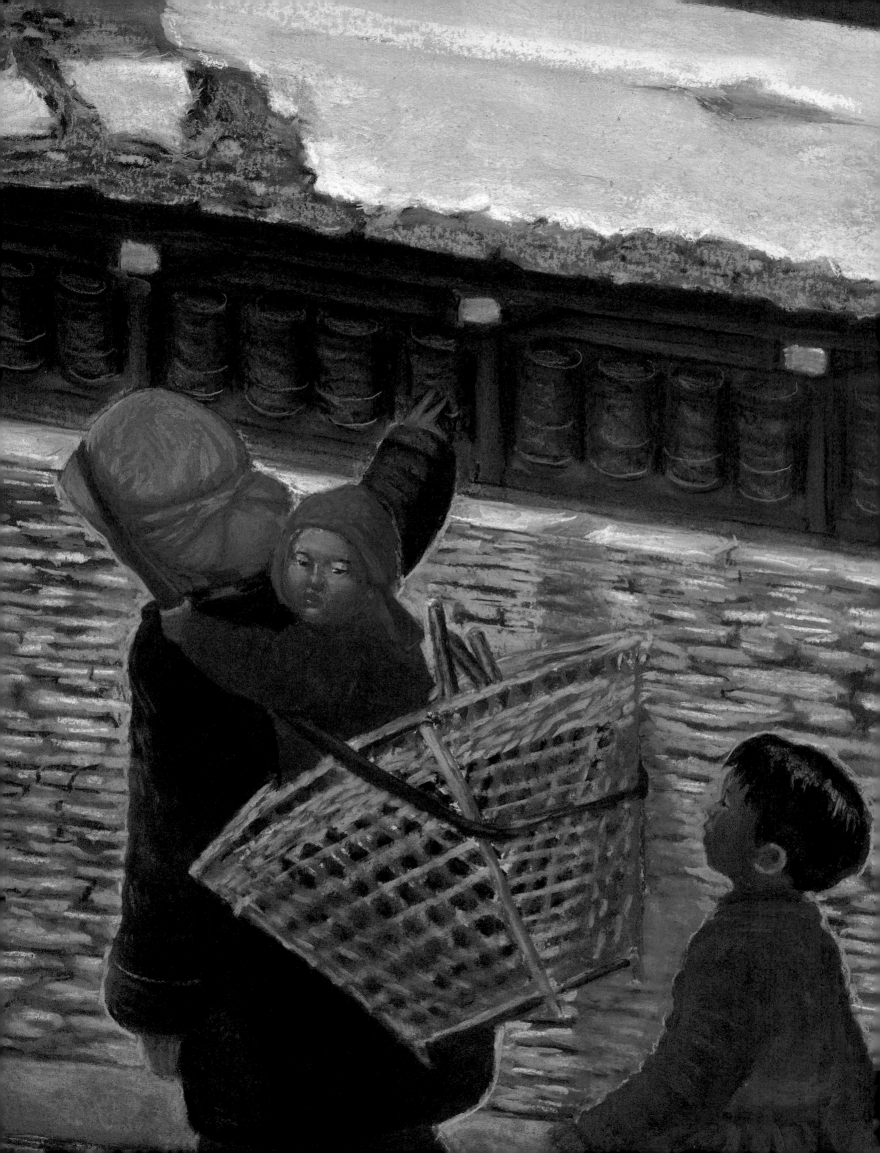

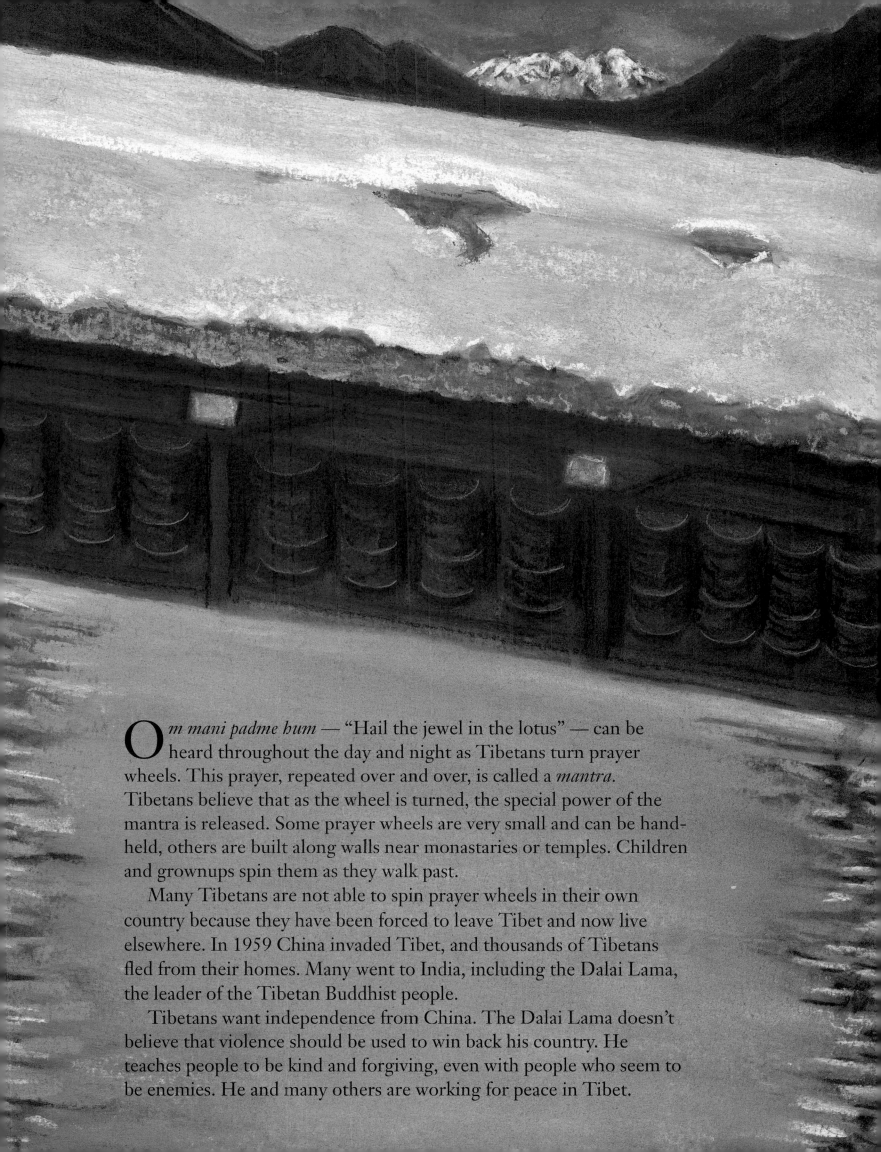

Om mani padme hum — "Hail the jewel in the lotus" — can be heard throughout the day and night as Tibetans turn prayer wheels. This prayer, repeated over and over, is called a *mantra*. Tibetans believe that as the wheel is turned, the special power of the mantra is released. Some prayer wheels are very small and can be hand-held, others are built along walls near monastaries or temples. Children and grownups spin them as they walk past.

Many Tibetans are not able to spin prayer wheels in their own country because they have been forced to leave Tibet and now live elsewhere. In 1959 China invaded Tibet, and thousands of Tibetans fled from their homes. Many went to India, including the Dalai Lama, the leader of the Tibetan Buddhist people.

Tibetans want independence from China. The Dalai Lama doesn't believe that violence should be used to win back his country. He teaches people to be kind and forgiving, even with people who seem to be enemies. He and many others are working for peace in Tibet.

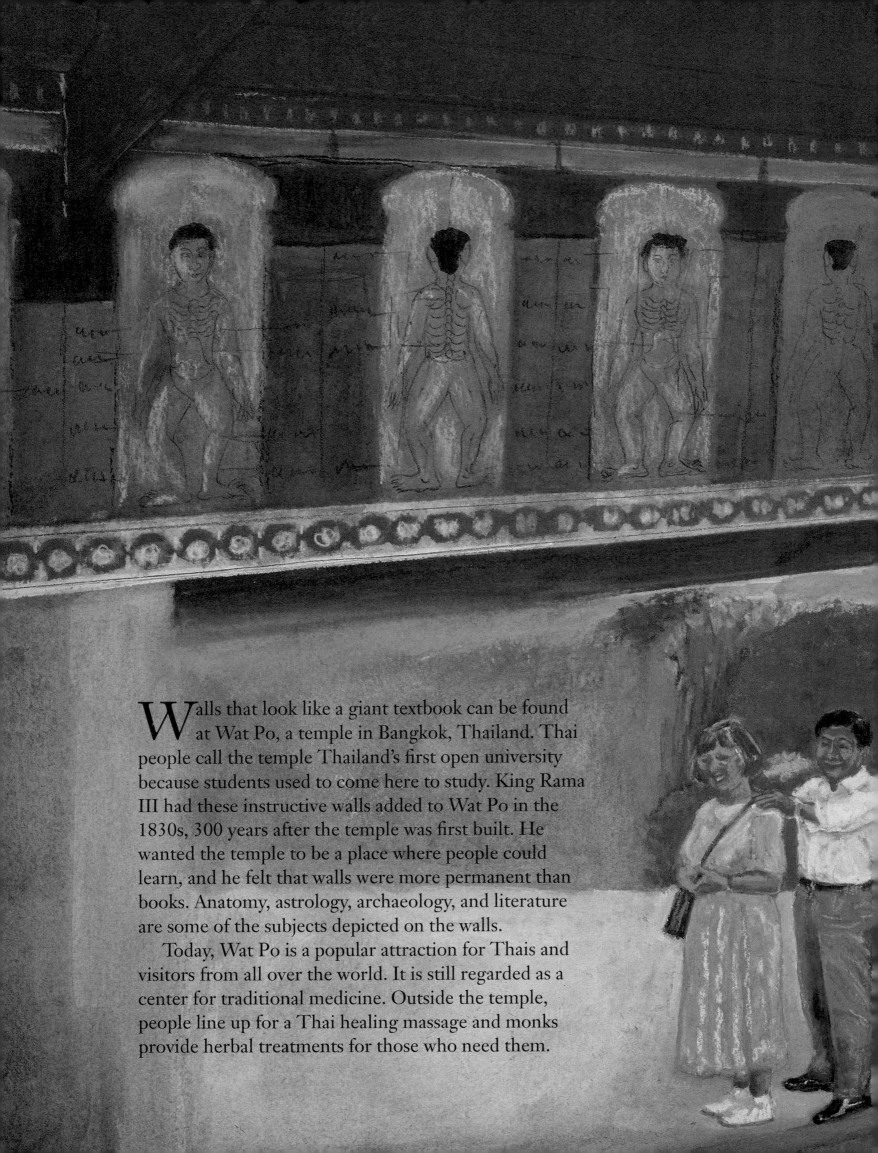

Walls that look like a giant textbook can be found at Wat Po, a temple in Bangkok, Thailand. Thai people call the temple Thailand's first open university because students used to come here to study. King Rama III had these instructive walls added to Wat Po in the 1830s, 300 years after the temple was first built. He wanted the temple to be a place where people could learn, and he felt that walls were more permanent than books. Anatomy, astrology, archaeology, and literature are some of the subjects depicted on the walls.

Today, Wat Po is a popular attraction for Thais and visitors from all over the world. It is still regarded as a center for traditional medicine. Outside the temple, people line up for a Thai healing massage and monks provide herbal treatments for those who need them.

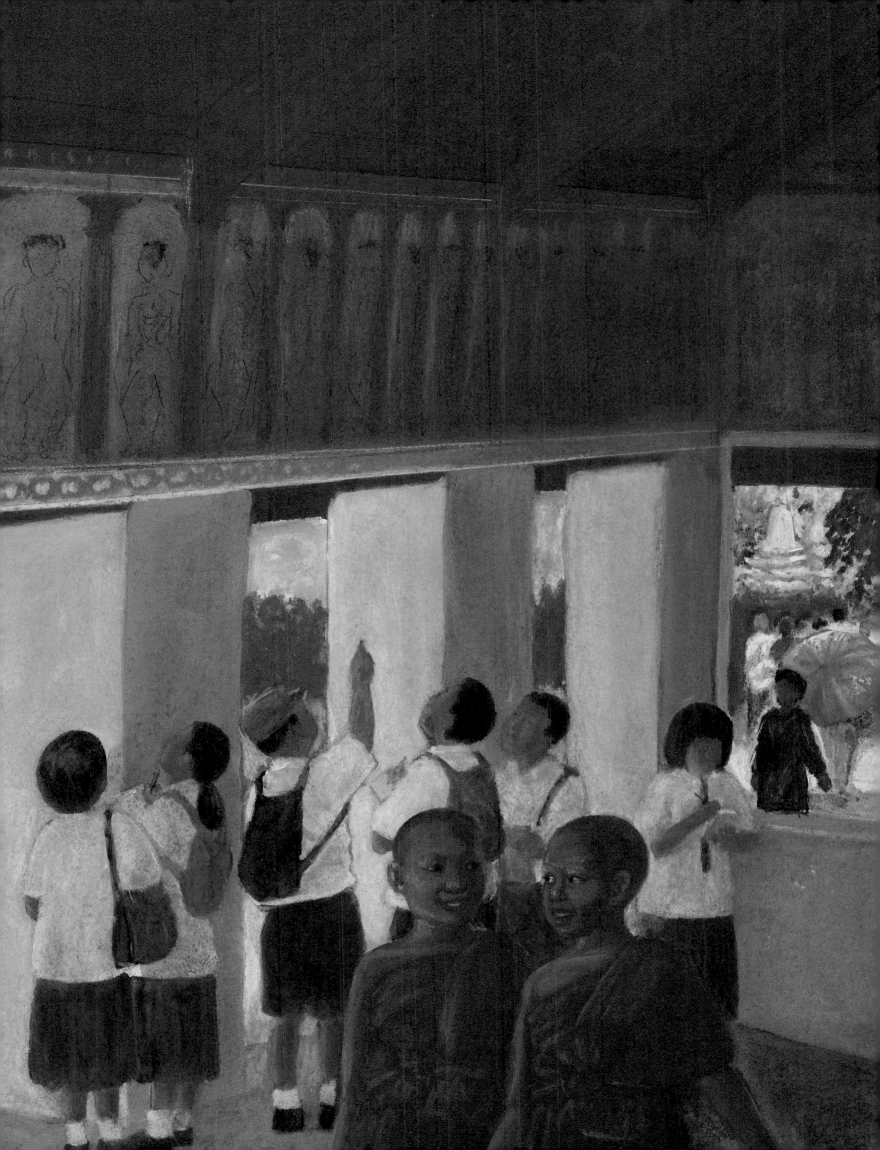

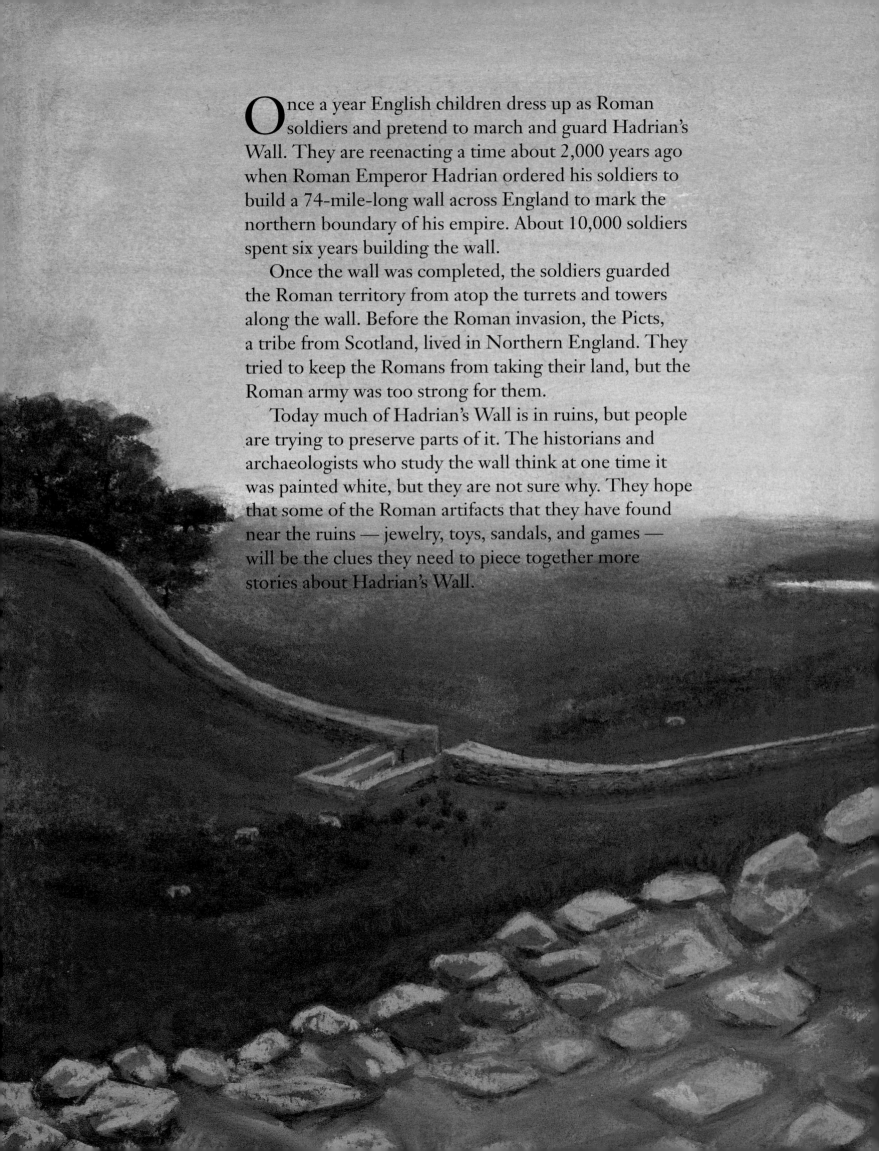

Once a year English children dress up as Roman soldiers and pretend to march and guard Hadrian's Wall. They are reenacting a time about 2,000 years ago when Roman Emperor Hadrian ordered his soldiers to build a 74-mile-long wall across England to mark the northern boundary of his empire. About 10,000 soldiers spent six years building the wall.

Once the wall was completed, the soldiers guarded the Roman territory from atop the turrets and towers along the wall. Before the Roman invasion, the Picts, a tribe from Scotland, lived in Northern England. They tried to keep the Romans from taking their land, but the Roman army was too strong for them.

Today much of Hadrian's Wall is in ruins, but people are trying to preserve parts of it. The historians and archaeologists who study the wall think at one time it was painted white, but they are not sure why. They hope that some of the Roman artifacts that they have found near the ruins — jewelry, toys, sandals, and games — will be the clues they need to piece together more stories about Hadrian's Wall.

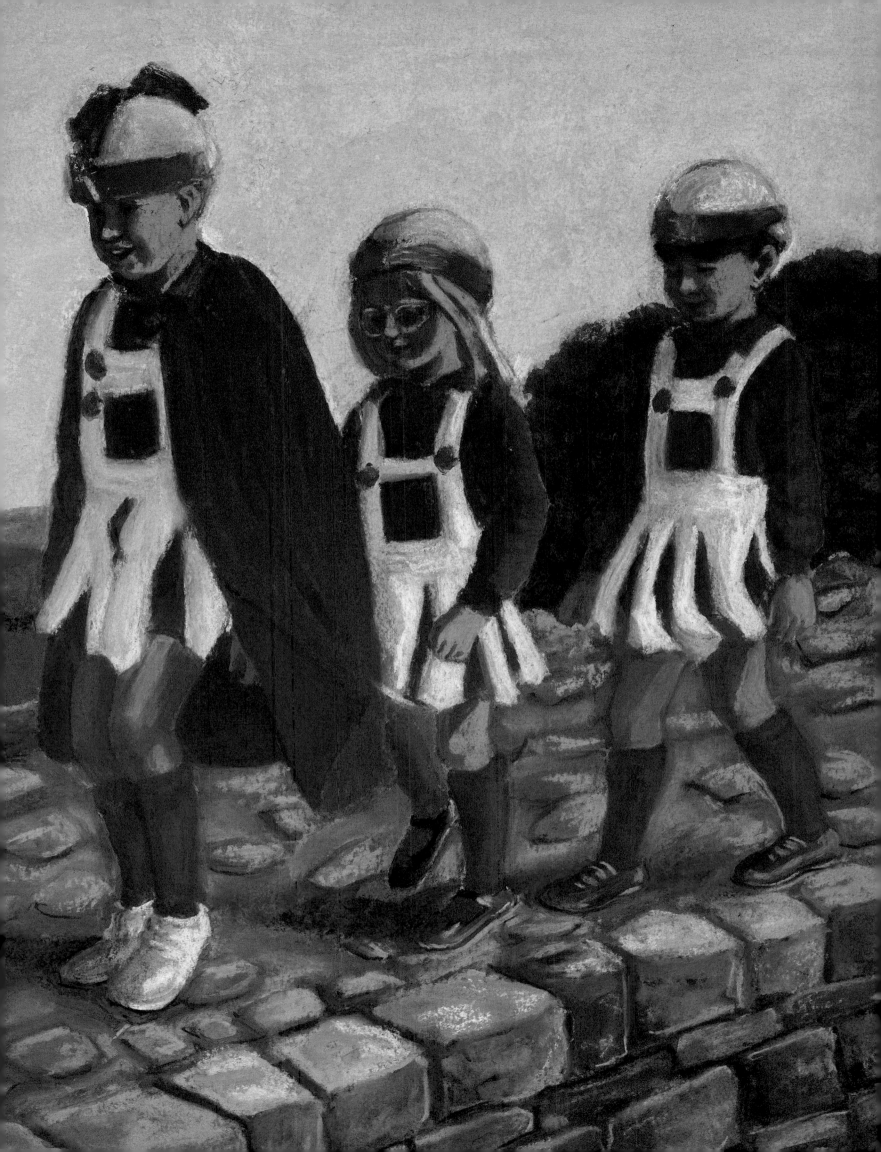

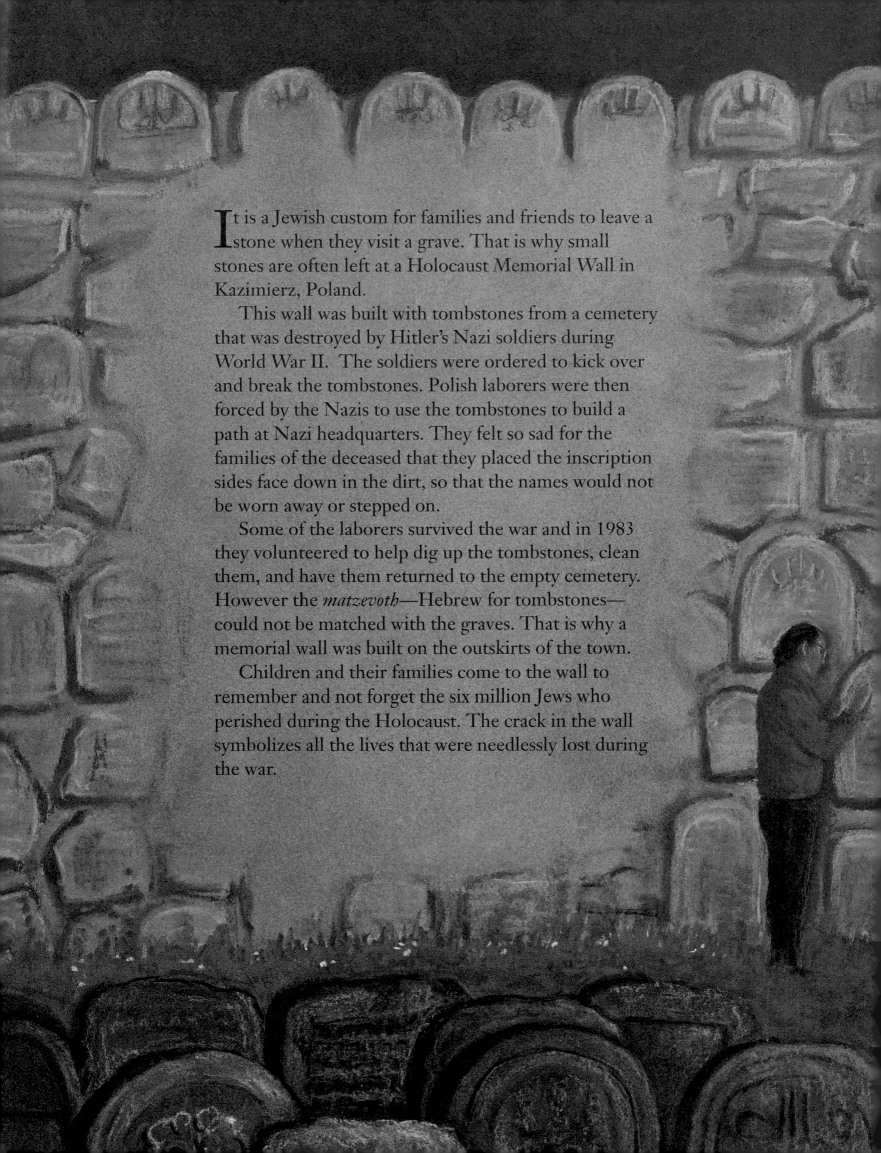

It is a Jewish custom for families and friends to leave a stone when they visit a grave. That is why small stones are often left at a Holocaust Memorial Wall in Kazimierz, Poland.

This wall was built with tombstones from a cemetery that was destroyed by Hitler's Nazi soldiers during World War II. The soldiers were ordered to kick over and break the tombstones. Polish laborers were then forced by the Nazis to use the tombstones to build a path at Nazi headquarters. They felt so sad for the families of the deceased that they placed the inscription sides face down in the dirt, so that the names would not be worn away or stepped on.

Some of the laborers survived the war and in 1983 they volunteered to help dig up the tombstones, clean them, and have them returned to the empty cemetery. However the *matzevoth*—Hebrew for tombstones—could not be matched with the graves. That is why a memorial wall was built on the outskirts of the town.

Children and their families come to the wall to remember and not forget the six million Jews who perished during the Holocaust. The crack in the wall symbolizes all the lives that were needlessly lost during the war.

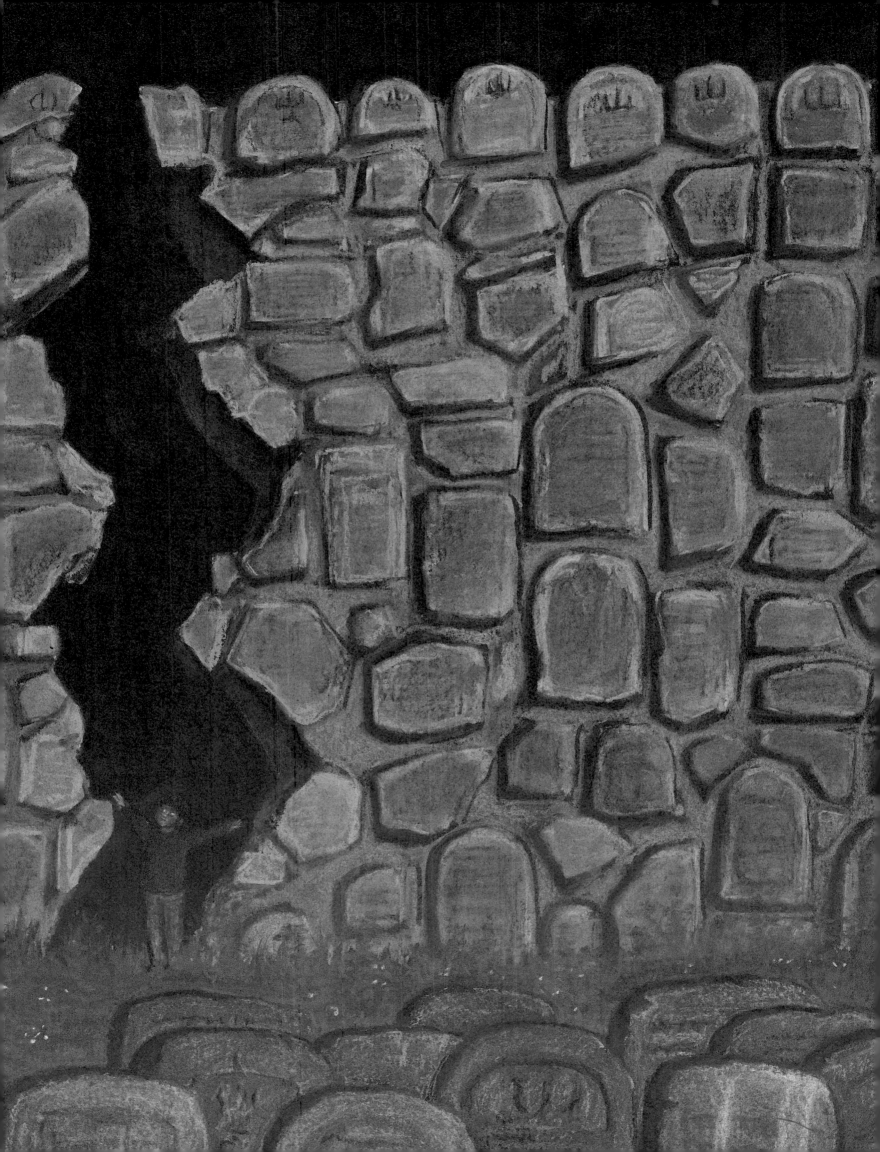

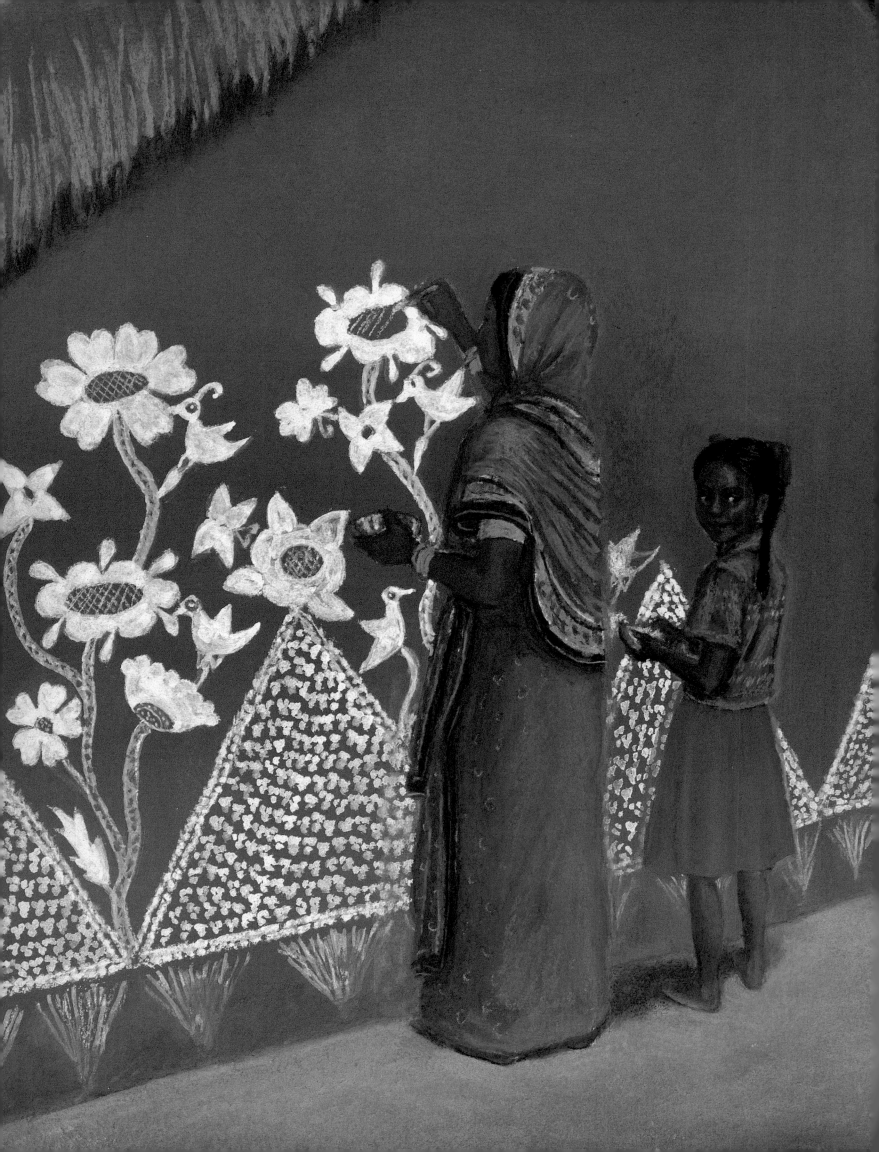

Many people in India believe Lakshmi's spirit will protect their home if they paint their walls during Divali, a Hindu festival of lights. Women and children please Lakshmi, the goddess of wealth and prosperity, by sketching peacocks, lotuses, and elephants on their walls with paint made from rice flour and water. A painting of a pyramid of rice, symbolic of the recent harvest, is often added to the wall.

During the evenings of this festival small oil lamps called *diyas* are lit to also honor Lakshmi. Divali is celebrated at the new moon that falls at the end of October or beginning of November; it marks the coming of the New Year for Hindus all over the world.

After Divali rain, wind, and sun fade the wall paintings. Every fall they are painted again.

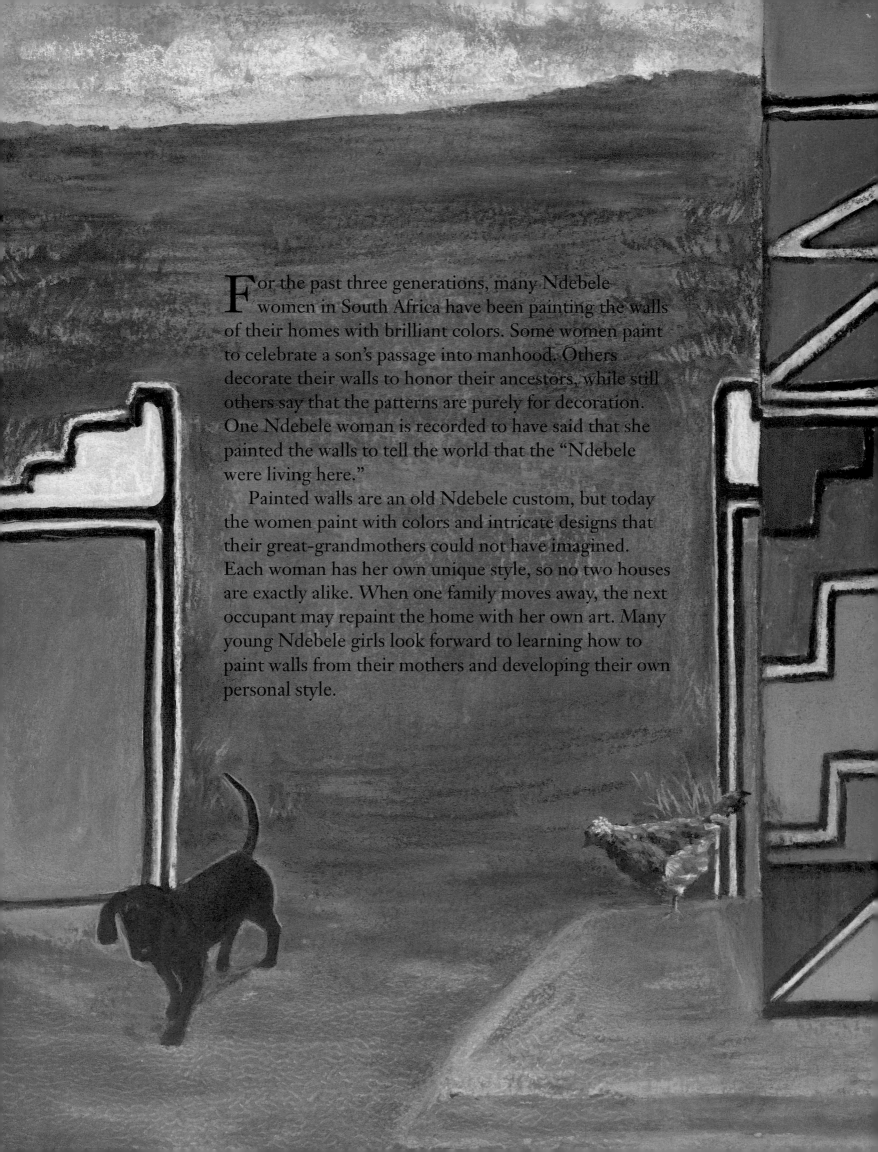

For the past three generations, many Ndebele women in South Africa have been painting the walls of their homes with brilliant colors. Some women paint to celebrate a son's passage into manhood. Others decorate their walls to honor their ancestors, while still others say that the patterns are purely for decoration. One Ndebele woman is recorded to have said that she painted the walls to tell the world that the "Ndebele were living here."

Painted walls are an old Ndebele custom, but today the women paint with colors and intricate designs that their great-grandmothers could not have imagined. Each woman has her own unique style, so no two houses are exactly alike. When one family moves away, the next occupant may repaint the home with her own art. Many young Ndebele girls look forward to learning how to paint walls from their mothers and developing their own personal style.

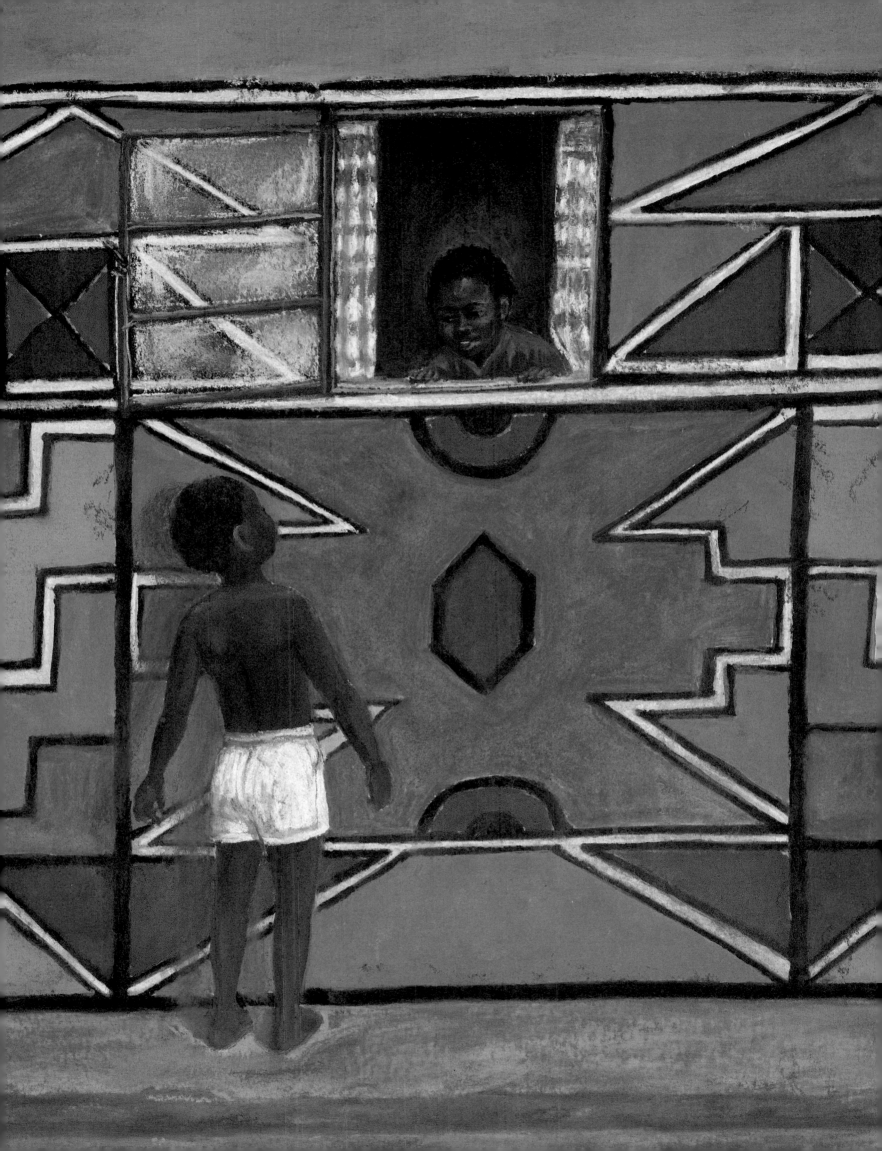

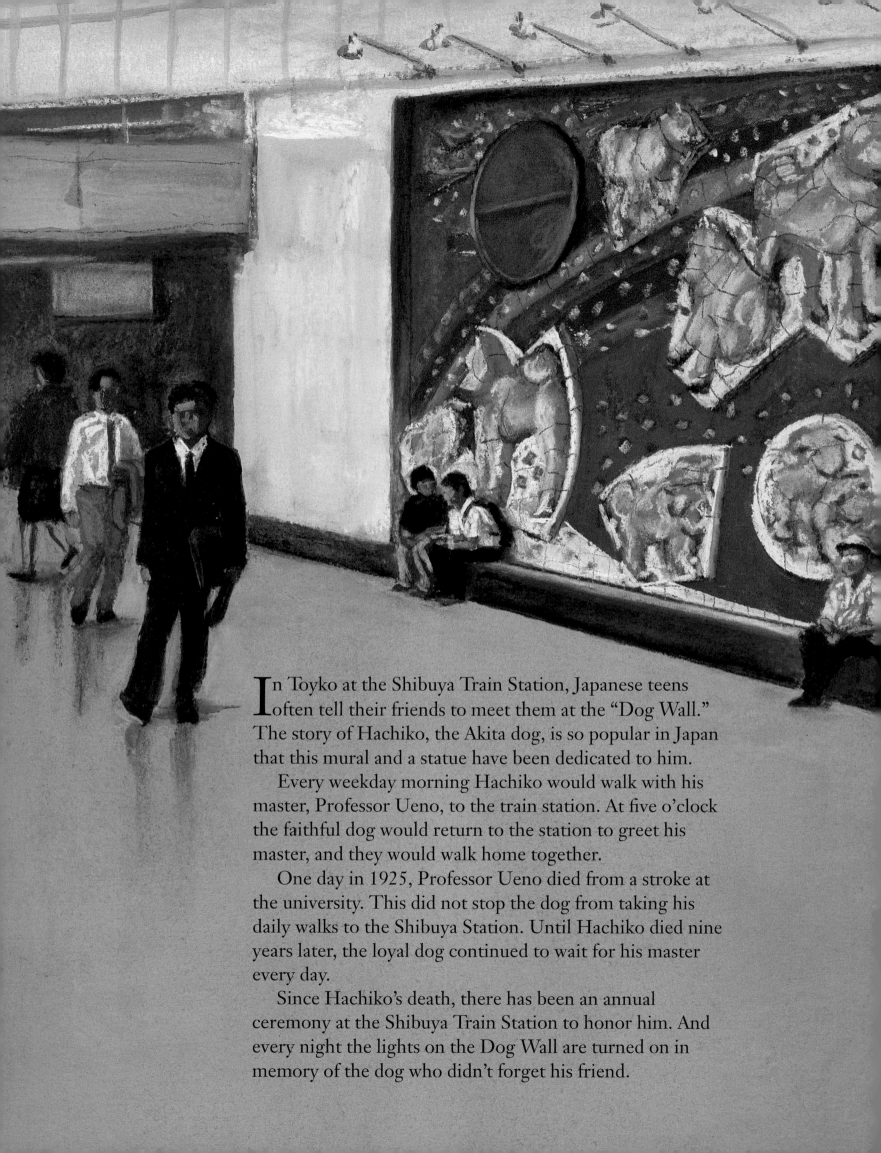

In Toyko at the Shibuya Train Station, Japanese teens often tell their friends to meet them at the "Dog Wall." The story of Hachiko, the Akita dog, is so popular in Japan that this mural and a statue have been dedicated to him.

Every weekday morning Hachiko would walk with his master, Professor Ueno, to the train station. At five o'clock the faithful dog would return to the station to greet his master, and they would walk home together.

One day in 1925, Professor Ueno died from a stroke at the university. This did not stop the dog from taking his daily walks to the Shibuya Station. Until Hachiko died nine years later, the loyal dog continued to wait for his master every day.

Since Hachiko's death, there has been an annual ceremony at the Shibuya Train Station to honor him. And every night the lights on the Dog Wall are turned on in memory of the dog who didn't forget his friend.

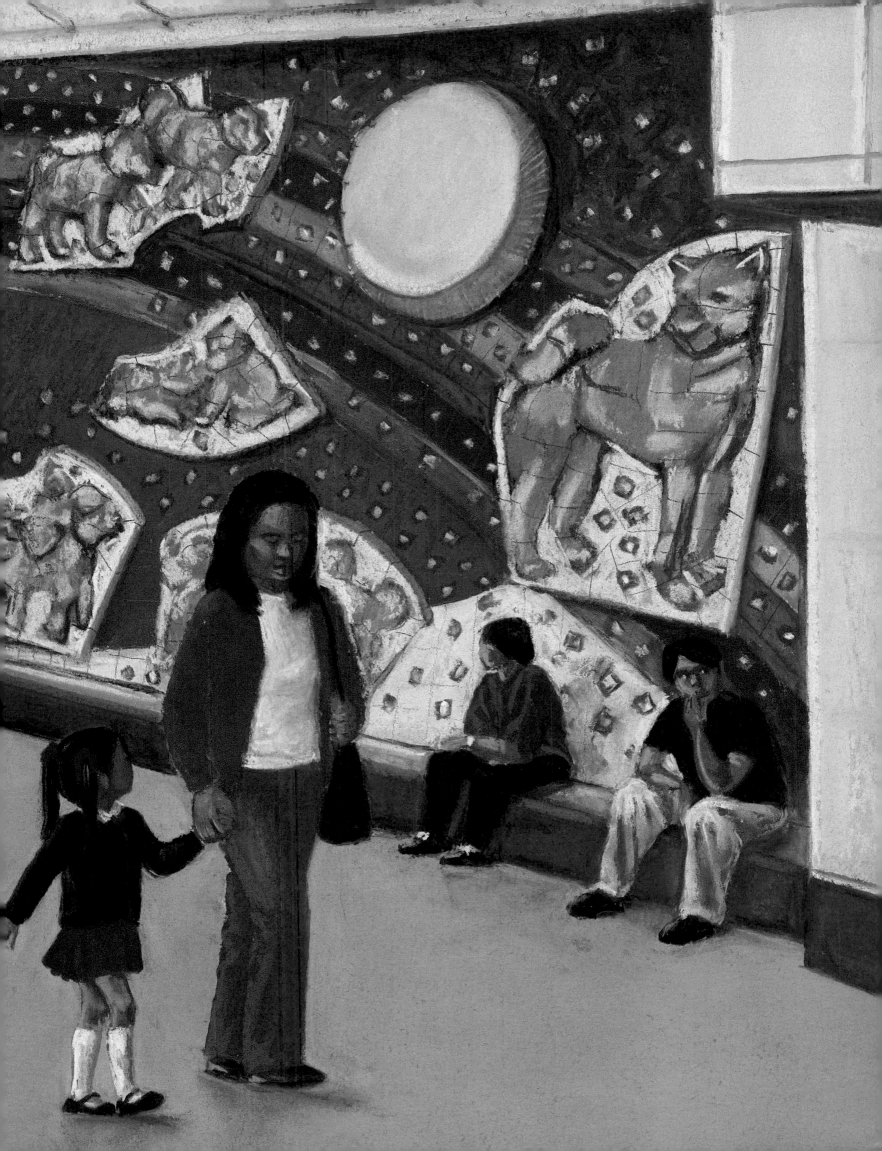

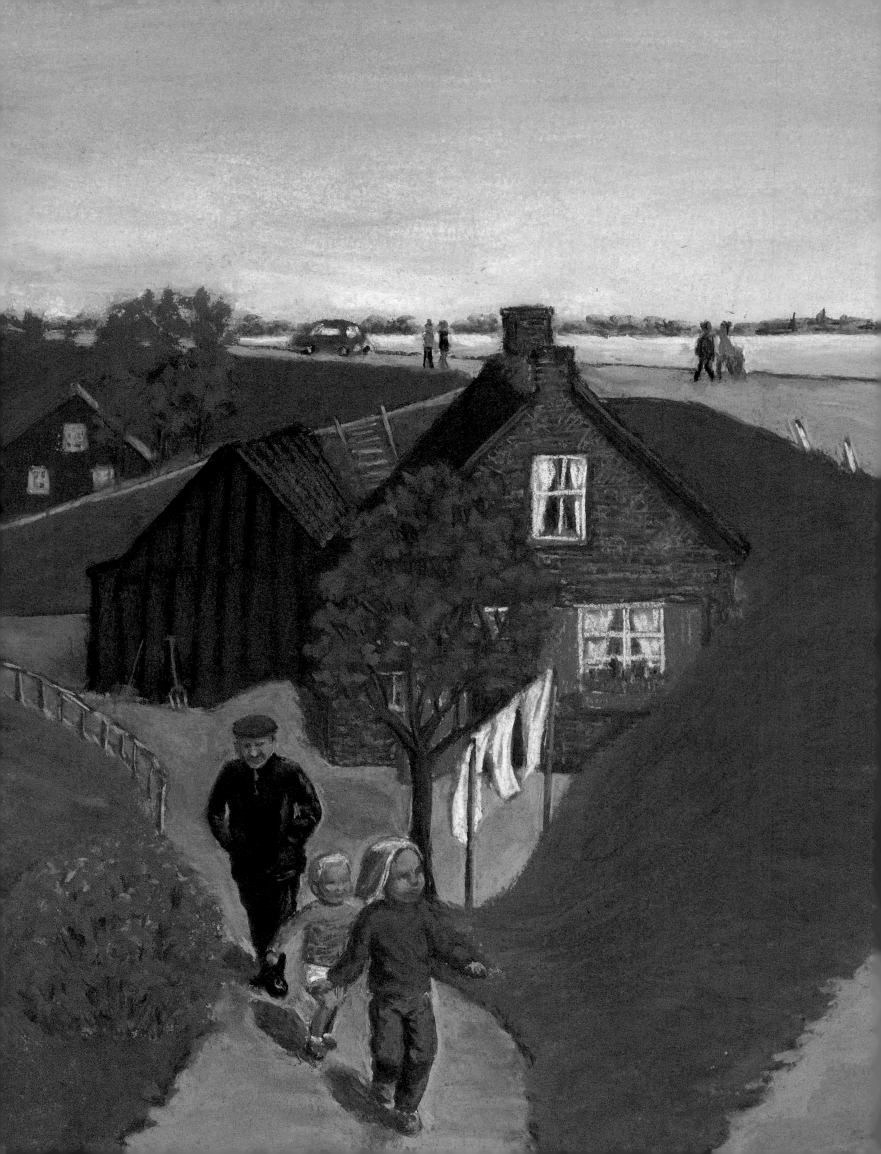

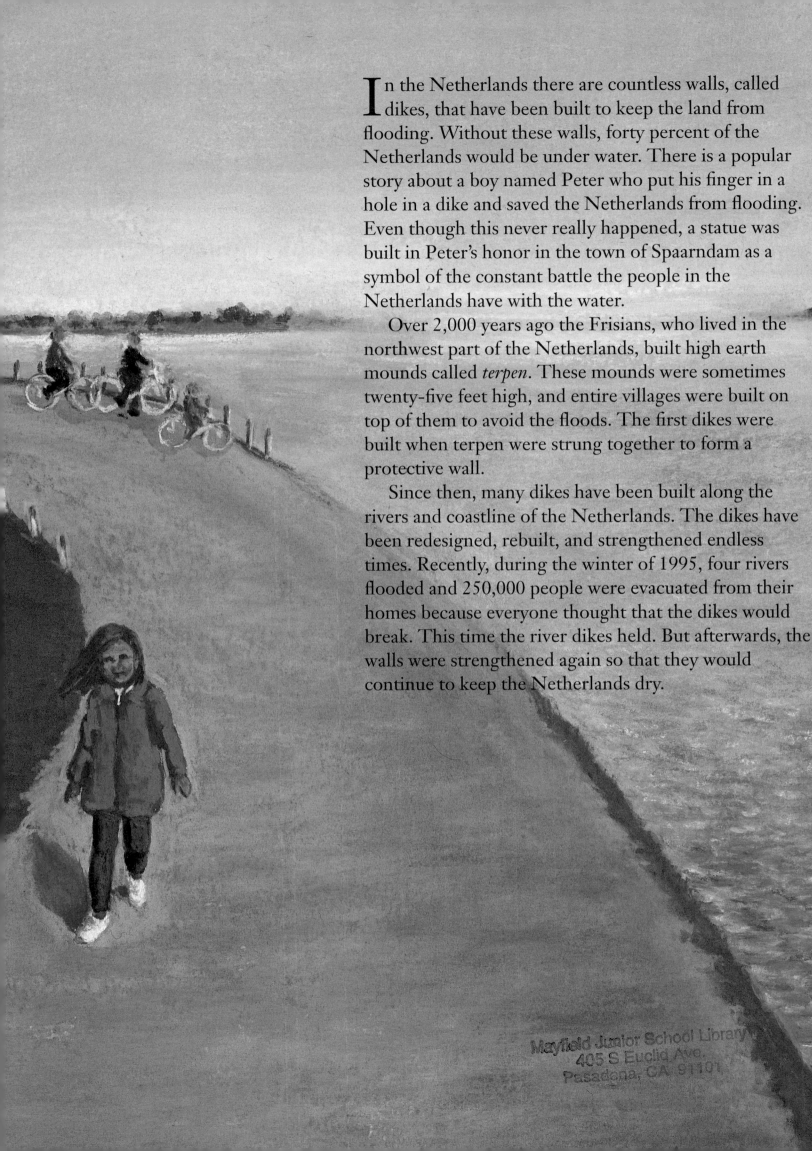

In the Netherlands there are countless walls, called dikes, that have been built to keep the land from flooding. Without these walls, forty percent of the Netherlands would be under water. There is a popular story about a boy named Peter who put his finger in a hole in a dike and saved the Netherlands from flooding. Even though this never really happened, a statue was built in Peter's honor in the town of Spaarndam as a symbol of the constant battle the people in the Netherlands have with the water.

Over 2,000 years ago the Frisians, who lived in the northwest part of the Netherlands, built high earth mounds called *terpen*. These mounds were sometimes twenty-five feet high, and entire villages were built on top of them to avoid the floods. The first dikes were built when terpen were strung together to form a protective wall.

Since then, many dikes have been built along the rivers and coastline of the Netherlands. The dikes have been redesigned, rebuilt, and strengthened endless times. Recently, during the winter of 1995, four rivers flooded and 250,000 people were evacuated from their homes because everyone thought that the dikes would break. This time the river dikes held. But afterwards, the walls were strengthened again so that they would continue to keep the Netherlands dry.

Mayfield Junior School Library
405 S Euclid Ave.
Pasadena, CA 91101

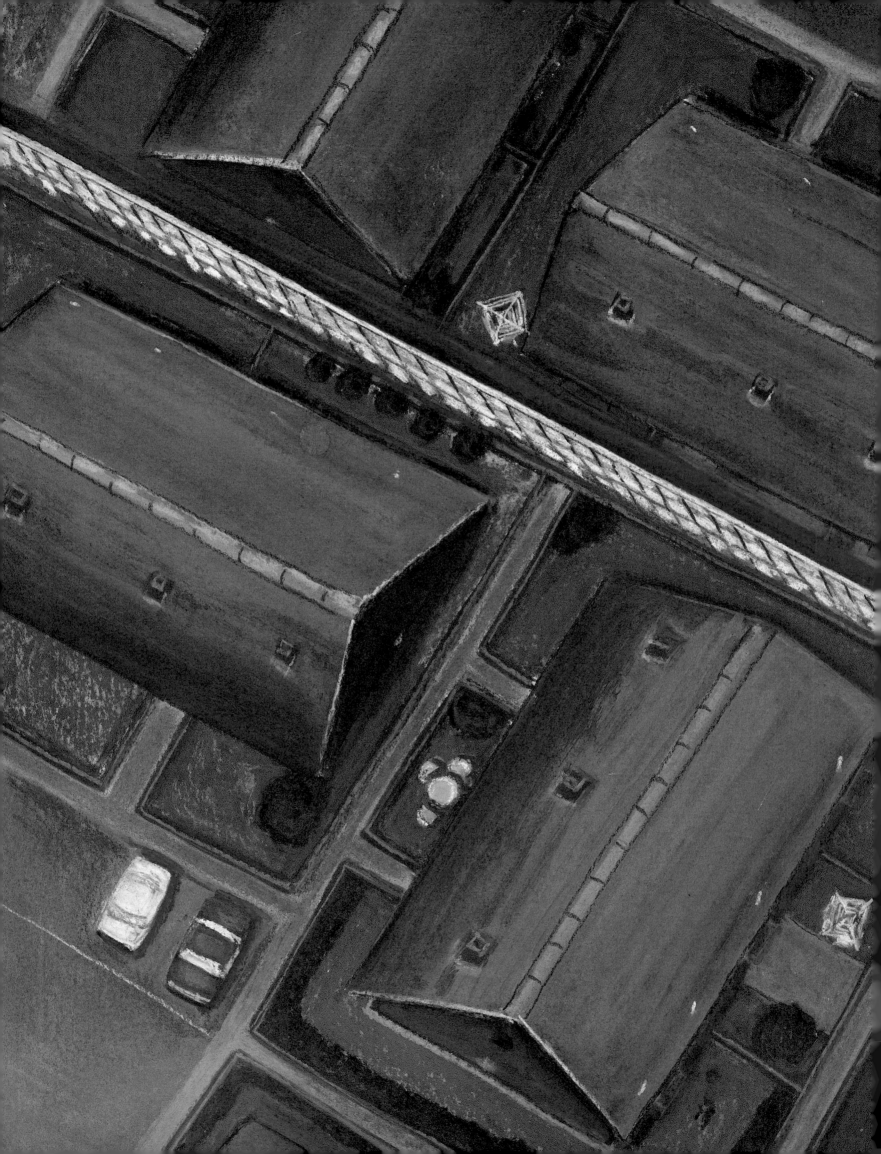

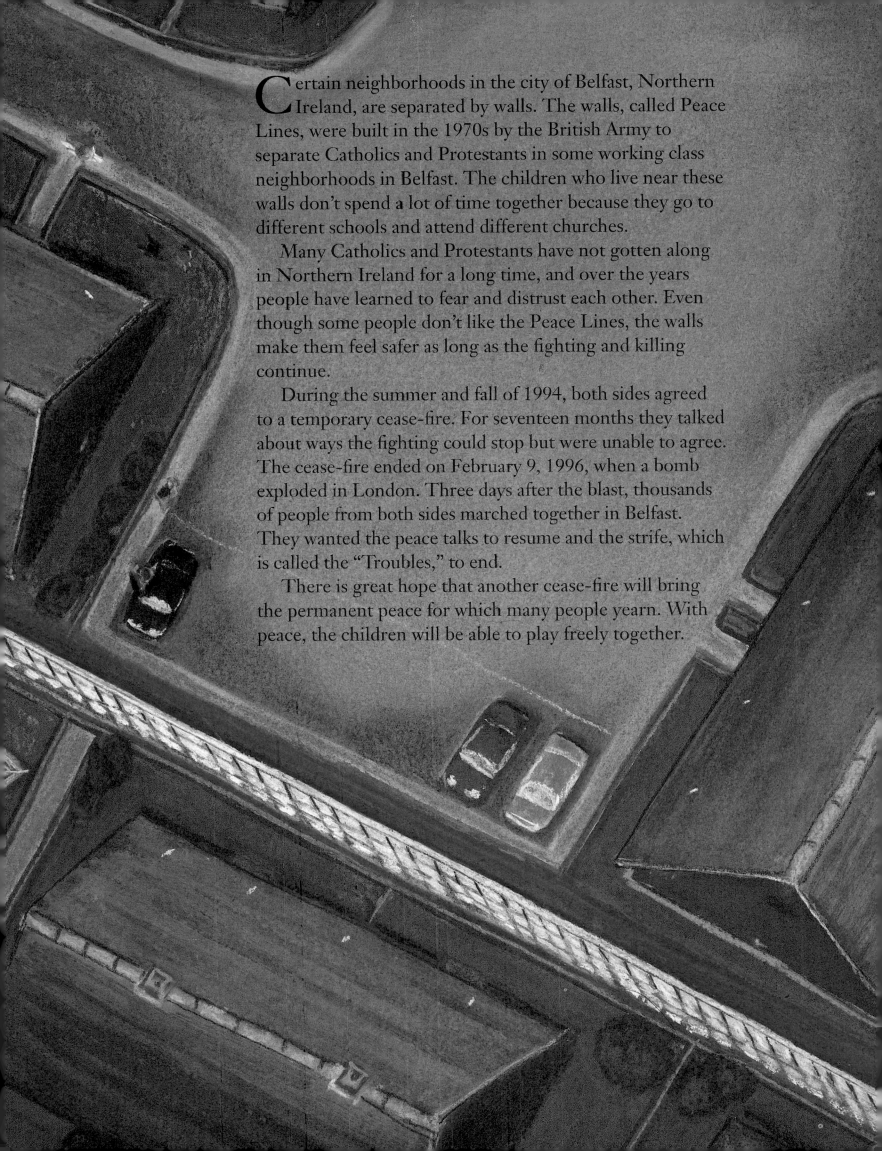

Certain neighborhoods in the city of Belfast, Northern Ireland, are separated by walls. The walls, called Peace Lines, were built in the 1970s by the British Army to separate Catholics and Protestants in some working class neighborhoods in Belfast. The children who live near these walls don't spend **a** lot of time together because they go to different schools and attend different churches.

Many Catholics and Protestants have not gotten along in Northern Ireland for a long time, and over the years people have learned to fear and distrust each other. Even though some people don't like the Peace Lines, the walls make them feel safer as long as the fighting and killing continue.

During the summer and fall of 1994, both sides agreed to a temporary cease-fire. For seventeen months they talked about ways the fighting could stop but were unable to agree. The cease-fire ended on February 9, 1996, when a bomb exploded in London. Three days after the blast, thousands of people from both sides marched together in Belfast. They wanted the peace talks to resume and the strife, which is called the "Troubles," to end.

There is great hope that another cease-fire will bring the permanent peace for which many people yearn. With peace, the children will be able to play freely together.

The Chinese poems carved into the barracks walls at Angel Island were saved by accident. These poems were written by Chinese immigrants who were lonely and angry. They were lonely because they missed their families in China, and they were angry because they were being held against their will at Angel Island, an immigration detention center in California's San Francisco Bay.

From 1910–1940, thousands of Chinese immigrants were detained at Angel Island because at that time the U.S. government had unfair laws for Chinese immigrants. Before allowing them into the country, U.S. officials asked the Chinese immigrants on Angel Island much harsher and stricter questions than the ones they asked European immigrants at Ellis Island, an immigration station near New York City.

Thirty years after the Angel Island Station closed, the barracks where many of these poems had been carved was going to be taken down. A park ranger noticed the Chinese writing on the walls, and he told people in the Chinese-American community about it. Thanks to him and the efforts of many others, the barracks was saved and turned into a museum. Today people go to Angel Island to read the poems and to listen to stories about the men, women, and children who were detained there.

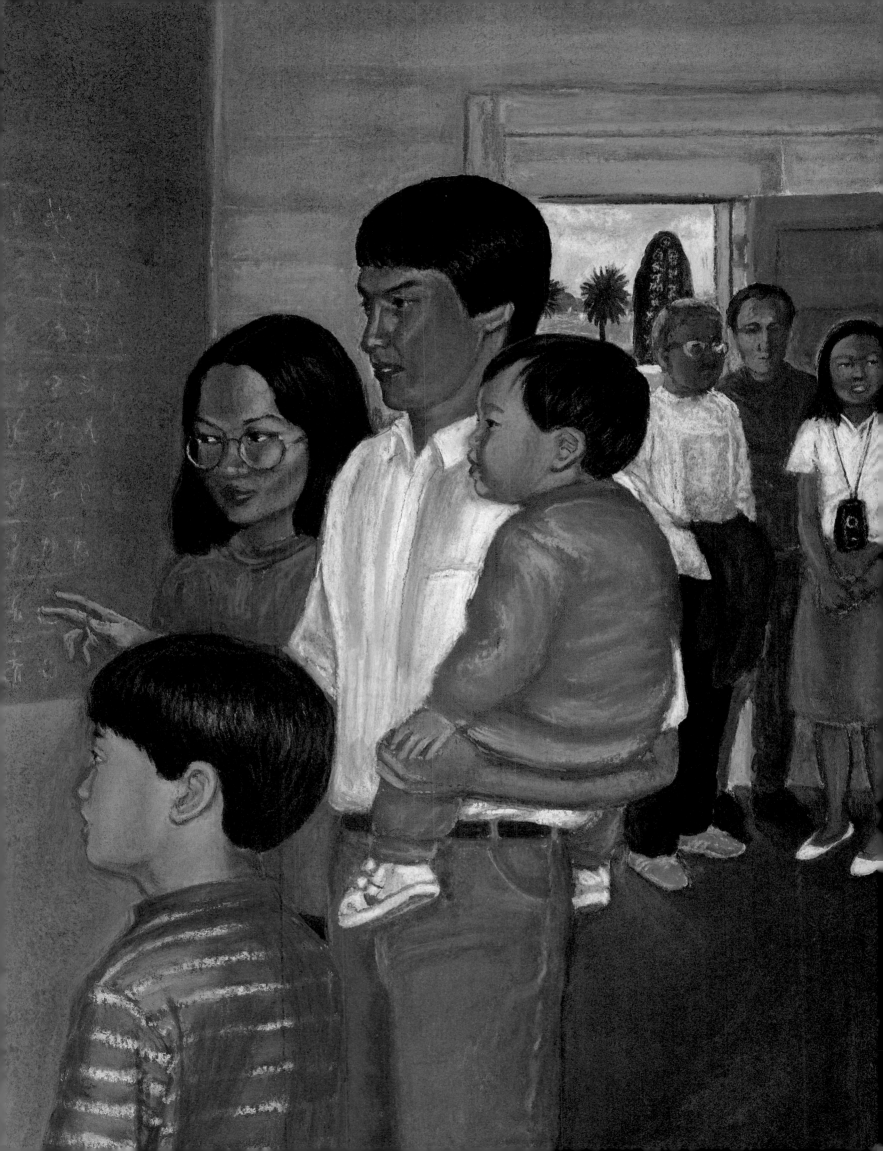

Thousands of messages have been written on the fence that surrounds the Isla Negra home of Chilean poet Pablo Neruda. Many of the messages praise and thank Neruda for writing beautiful poetry and for speaking out for human rights.

Neruda didn't like it when a military government took over his country on September 11, 1973. A few weeks later he died, and the new military leader of Chile warned people to stay away from Neruda's home. However, for seventeen years people came secretly to write on the fence of the poet who as a child was known to say he was "hunting for poems."

When he was ten, Neruda showed one of his poems to his father. The father was so surprised by the beautiful words that he asked his son who really wrote the poem. Neruda's father thought that his son spent too much time writing poetry, and Pablo's schoolmates often made fun of him. But Pablo couldn't stop writing, and at thirteen, his first poems were published. Three years later, he took the pen name Pablo Neruda. He chose Neruda after one of his favorite Czechoslovakian poets.

Today, the government of Chile is freely elected and is proud of Neruda's legacy. Neruda's admirers continue to visit his home to write tributes to the boy who grew up to become one of the greatest poets in the world.

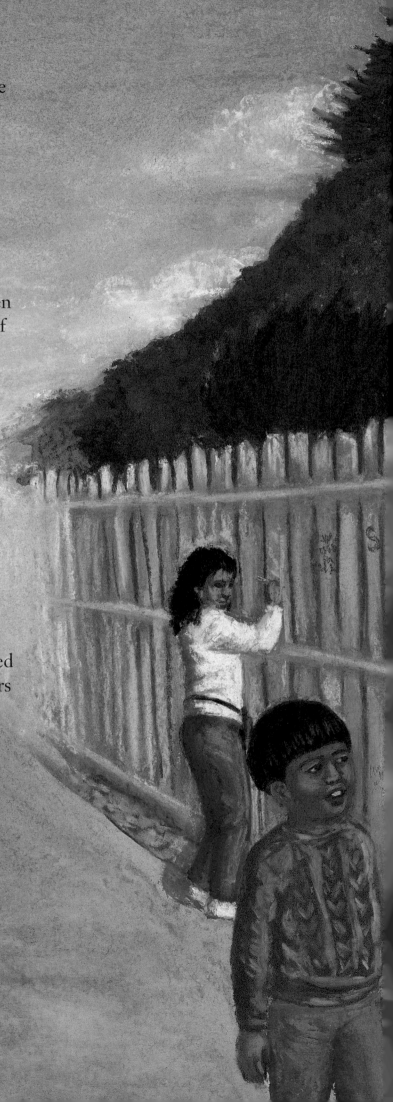

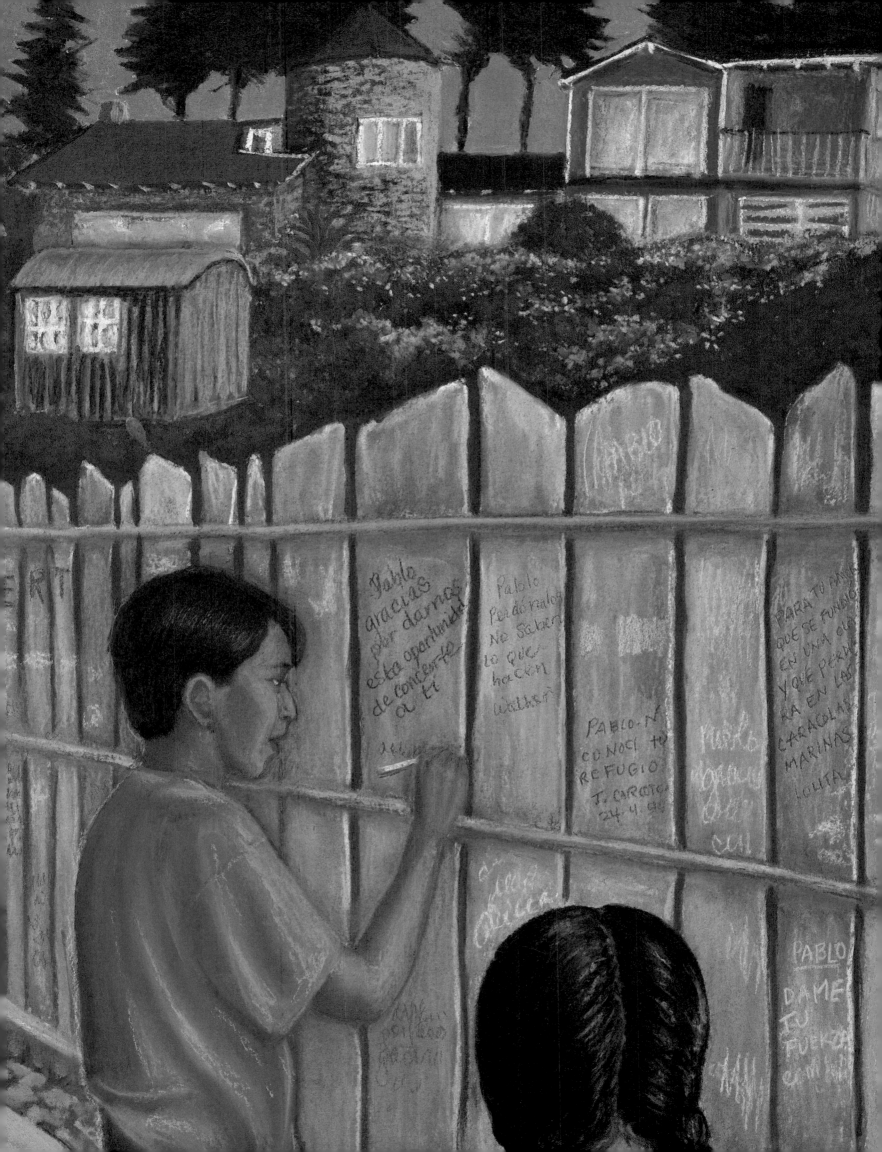

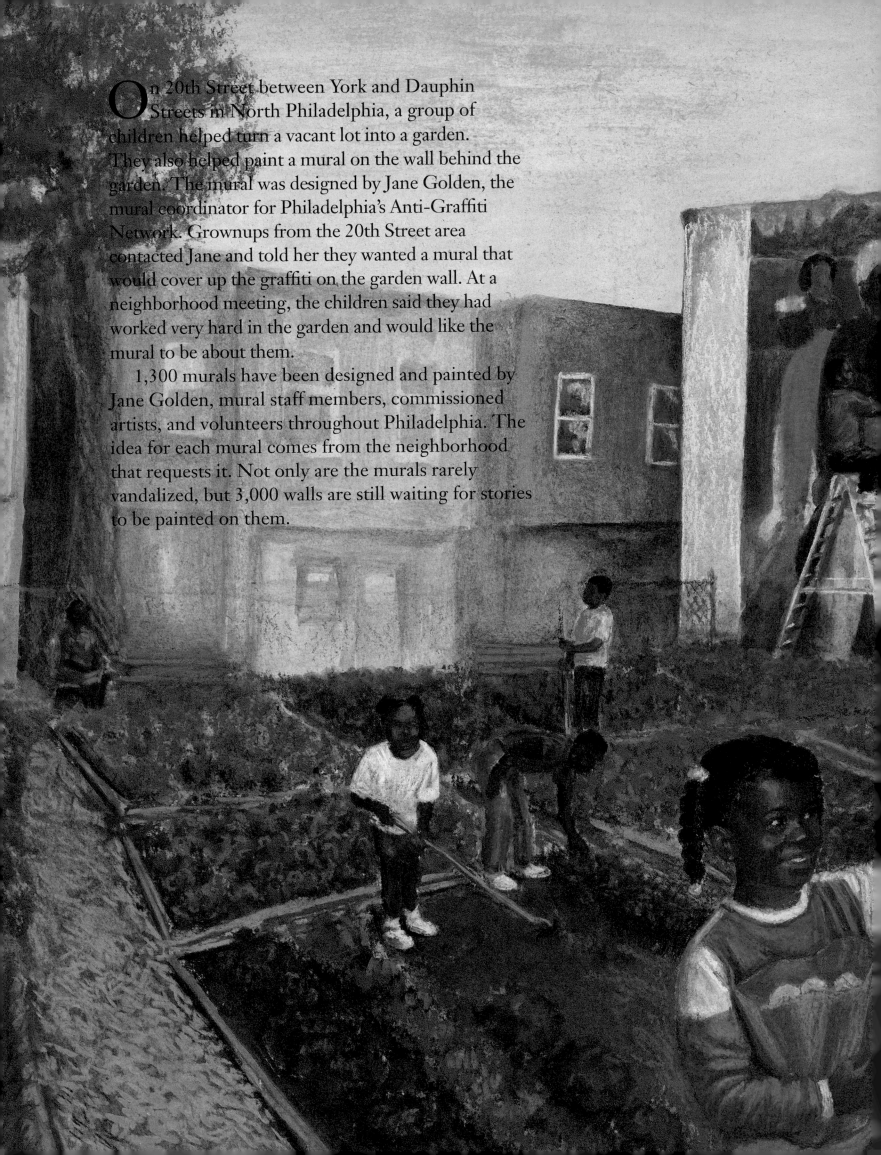

On 20th Street between York and Dauphin Streets in North Philadelphia, a group of children helped turn a vacant lot into a garden. They also helped paint a mural on the wall behind the garden. The mural was designed by Jane Golden, the mural coordinator for Philadelphia's Anti-Graffiti Network. Grownups from the 20th Street area contacted Jane and told her they wanted a mural that would cover up the graffiti on the garden wall. At a neighborhood meeting, the children said they had worked very hard in the garden and would like the mural to be about them.

1,300 murals have been designed and painted by Jane Golden, mural staff members, commissioned artists, and volunteers throughout Philadelphia. The idea for each mural comes from the neighborhood that requests it. Not only are the murals rarely vandalized, but 3,000 walls are still waiting for stories to be painted on them.

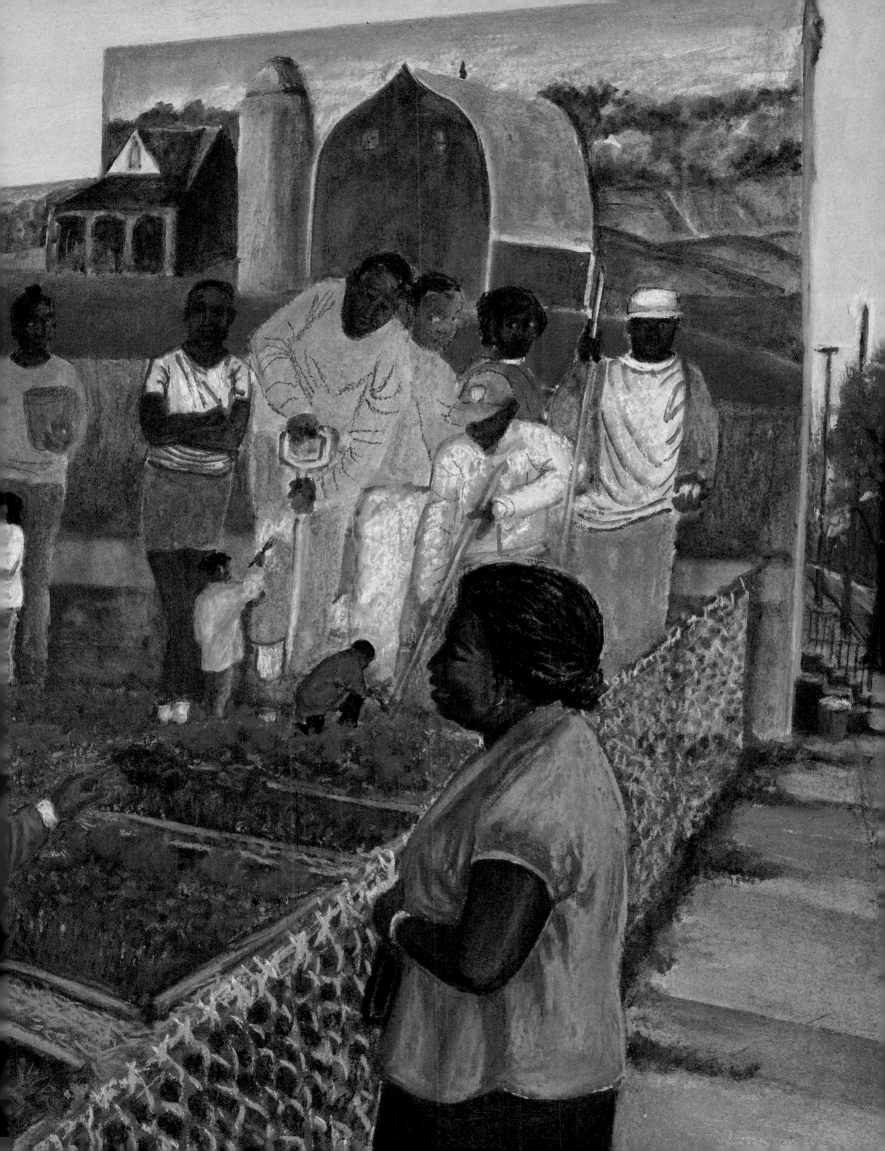

For Dianne Webb.
Thanks for listening to my stories.
— MBK

For O.B.
Footing, mortar, and foundation.
— ASO

1,2 Endleaves

The front endleaves show a portion of Stena Mira, The Peace Wall, in Russia, where messages of peace have been hand-painted by Latvian, Russian, Canadian and American children. The wall was built in 1990 — a year after the Berlin Wall was taken down — on the old Arbat, a busy pedestrian street in Moscow.

In 1993 a similar wall, the Friendship Wall (shown on the back endleaves), was built by K-8 students at the Union School in Union, Maine, after several teachers returned from a trip to Moscow.

3 Cover

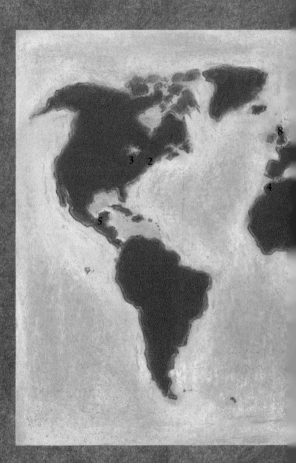

In November of 1993, Annie and I were Visiting Artists at an elementary school in Indianapolis, Indiana. We were walking down the hall when Cathy Clady, a third grade teacher, stopped us to tell us about her husband, Kent Clady, a sixth grade teacher at the John Marshall Middle School. She said that he used our first book, *Talking Walls* (Tilbury House, Publishers, 1992), in his social studies class, and that his students did an entire unit on walls which included fixing up the entrance wall of an apartment complex near the school.

The sixth graders worked hard, scraping and painting the wall. The residents of the apartment complex were so pleased with the students' work that they contacted local T.V. stations and even invited the sixth graders to use their pool at the end of the year for a cookout. After I returned home, I wrote to Kent Clady and asked him to send me slides of his students at work on the wall. I have shown these slides and told the story of the "repaired wall" countless times to teachers throughout the country.

During the fall of 1995 and winter of 1996, we worked on cover ideas for *Talking Walls: The Stories Continue.* Annie wanted to draw children doing something at a wall, and we decided that the sixth graders in Indiana and their wall project would make a great cover.

4 Fez

Fez is really three different cities in one. Fez de Bali is the old city with the medina. Fez Jedid also has its own wall and the Royal Palace where the King of Morocco stays when he visits. Modern Fez is known as the Ville Nouvelle, or new city. Rabat, also a walled city, has been the capital of Morocco since 1912.

There are many walled cities around the world. Some of them are Kabul in Afghanistan, York in England, Jerusalem in Israel, Londonderry in Northern Ireland, and Chiang Mai in Thailand. In Manila, in the Philippines, Intramuros is the oldest part of the city. *Intramuros* means "inside the walls" in Spanish.

5 Bonampak

In 1946 in the dense forest of the Eastern Chiapas Mountains in Mexico, three rooms of magnificent wall murals painted over a thousand years ago were discovered by Maya scholars. They named the paintings the Murals of Bonampak. Bonampak means "painted wall" in Mayan. Maya murals can also be seen in many other locations such as Chichén Itzá, Mexico. These murals are also fading, but they are not as old as those in Bonampak. Reproductions of the Bonampak murals can be seen at the Peabody Museum at Harvard University in Cambridge, Massachusetts, and in two museums in Mexico.

6 Prayer Wheels

Tenzin Gyatso is the fourteenth Dalai Lama. Tibetan Buddhists believe that when the thirteenth Dalai Lama died in 1933, he was reincarnated as a child.

Lamas went to look for this child and took a rosary with them that had belonged to the thirteenth Dalai Lama. They were told that a special child lived in a turquoise house, so they disguised themselves as servants and went to visit the boy. The two-year-old child saw the rosary and said, "This is mine." He was also able to pick out many objects on a table that belonged to the former Dalai Lama. At age four, with his parents' blessings, the young boy went to live with the lamas in Lhasa, Tibet, where they took good care of him and taught him how to be a lama.

At the age of fifteen, in 1950, he became the fourteenth Dalai Lama. The term *lama* means teacher, and *dalai* is the Mongolian word for ocean. For his teaching of kindness and peace, the Dalai Lama was awarded the Nobel Peace Prize in 1989.

7 Wat Po

Wat Po is also called Wat Pra Jetupon. The oldest and largest temple in Bangkok, it was built in the sixteenth century. Today there are sixteen gates in the complex, but only a few are open to the public. The complex includes living quarters for monks, many religious buildings, and an enormous statue of a reclining Buddha. The statue is 150 feet long and entirely covered with gold leaf.

8 Hadrian's Wall

The Romans called the people living in Northern England Picts because they painted their skin. The Picts fought the Romans for many years. After Hadrian's death in A.D. 138, Emperor Antonius built a 40-mile-long wall 100 miles north of Hadrian's Wall. But it was abandoned after only twenty years of occupation, and Hadrian's Wall once again marked the Northern boundary for the Roman Empire.

English Heritage, a London-based organization, is responsible for preserving Hadrian's Wall. Every ten years people gather to walk along the seventy-four miles of the wall and its ruins. These walks were begun in 1849 and only suspended during both World Wars. The next pilgrimage, set for 1999, is being planned now.

9 Kazimierz

On September 1, 1939, German Chancellor Adolph Hilter invaded Poland and within weeks took over most of the country. Over the next few years every Jewish community in Poland was destroyed and three million Jews were murdered. Only about 5,000 Jews live in Poland today.

There are nearly 2,100 Jewish memorials in Poland that memorialize the victims of the Holocaust. Tens of thousands of Jews from Israel, Western Europe, and the United States visit Poland every year.

At the Holocaust Memorial Museum in Washington, D.C., a Wall of Remembrance was built as a memorial to the children who were murdered during the Holocaust. The tiles used to build the wall were handpainted by children from throughout the U.S.

10 Divali (also Diwali or Dipavali)

Divali means "garland of lights." Painting walls to honor Lakshmi is just one aspect of this Hindu holiday.

During Divali, Hindus also light diyas to celebrate the story of the return of Sita and Rama to their kingdom. Their story is very exciting and is told often during Divali. Prince Rama and his wife Sita had been banished from their home by the king. For fourteen years they lived happily in the forest with Lakshman, Rama's brother, until Sita was kidnapped by the ten-headed demon Ravana. Rama rescued Sita with the help of Hanuman, the monkey general, and Ravana was killed. The diyas were lit to guide Sita and Rama back to their kingdom. Once home, Rama was crowned king.

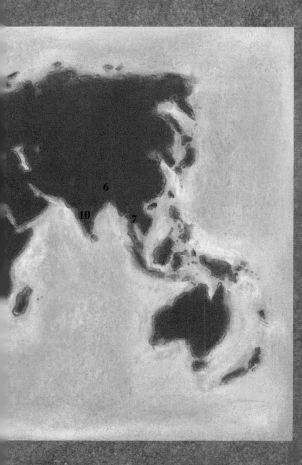

11 Ndebele

Before the 1940s the Ndebele (en-de bĕ'lē), one of many ethnic groups in South Africa, decorated their walls simply with earth pigments. Bluing was added once it became available. Today the wall decorations change as life changes in South Africa. Earth pigments are still used, along with many colors of commercial paint.

Across South Africa, Ndebele families today live in many kinds of housing, from high-rise city apartments to thatched-roof homes in rural areas. Not all Ndebele homes are painted.

12 Hachiko

The Japanese consider the Akita dog to be a national treasure. They regard it as a loyal friend and a symbol of good health. Originally it was bred as a hunting dog in the mountains of northern Japan. Small statues of Akita are often given to a new baby in hopes that the infant will have a happy, healthy life. Helen Keller introduced the Akita to the United States after she was given a dog as a present while vising Japan.

13 Dikes

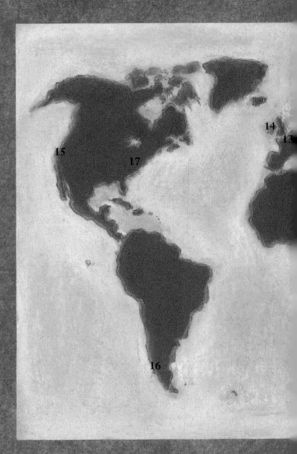

In the United States dikes are often called levees. "Levee" comes from the French word *lever*, which means "to raise." Levees are usually made of sandbags and banked-up earth. About 2,200 miles of them have been built along the southern part of the Mississippi River. The first levee on the Mississippi was built in New Orleans in 1718 to keep the river from flooding some fertile land. It was only three feet high. Today levees are fifteen to thirty feet high.

14 Peace Lines

Since 1969 about 3,000 people have died as a result of the Troubles in Belfast. People have a hard time agreeing on the reasons for the Troubles. The *Nationalists* support a United Ireland, and *Unionists* support continuing to be part of the United Kingdom. There are many people in Northern Ireland who support neither group because they feel each one is too extreme.

Another divided city is Nicosia in Cyprus. Turkey invaded Cyprus in 1974 and occupied the northern half of it. As the result of this war, there is a demarcation line that cuts through the middle of Nicosia, the capital of Cyprus. The Greeks live on the south side of the city, and the Turks live on the north side.

15 Angel Island

From 1910–1940, Angel Island was the port of entry for an estimated 175,000 Chinese immigrants. It was modeled after New York's Ellis Island and used as a detention site for Chinese waiting to pass physicals and have immigration papers accepted. Twenty-five percent of the Chinese were refused entry. By comparison, only two percent of the immigrants who traveled to Ellis Island were refused entry. Even though the average stay was two to three weeks, many detainees stayed on Angel Island for up to three years. On Ellis Island, the average stay was about five hours, although some arrivals had to stay longer because they had contagious diseases.

16 Pablo Neruda

Neruda was awarded the Nobel Prize for Literature in 1971. His birth name was Neftali Ricardo Reyes Basoalto. He was greatly influenced by Gabriela Mistral, another Chilean poet, who was the first woman in Latin America to be awarded the Nobel Prize for Literature (1945).

Neruda died of a heart attack and cancer in 1973, but many thought that he really died from a broken heart. President Salvatore Allende, his close friend, was assasinated by the followers of General Pinochet in a military coup d'état two weeks before Neruda's death. After Allende's assasination, many of Neruda's colleagues were imprisoned or killed by the new dictator.

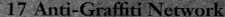

17 Anti-Graffiti Network

The Anti-Graffiti Network started in 1983. Wilson Goode, Philadelphia's first African-American mayor, promised to help reduce the amount of graffiti in the city. He decided to work closely with the young people involved in doing the wall-writing, channeling their negative behavior into something positive. Young people who are caught writing graffiti are asked to clean it off or attend art classes where they can learn to use their skills to help create murals. Rachel Bagby and Willi Mae Clark were two of the adults in the 20th Street neighborhood who helped with the garden mural. Children who attend the Pratt and Duckrey Schools in North Philadelphia suggested the garden mural for our book.

Across the continent in Chemainus, a small coastal town in British Columbia, Canada, another mural project is taking place. Since 1983, murals that tell stories of the town's history have been painted on the walls by artists. Chemainus is known as the "Little Town That Did," because the murals have revitalized the town. They attract thousands of visitors every year who travel there to look at the stories on the walls.

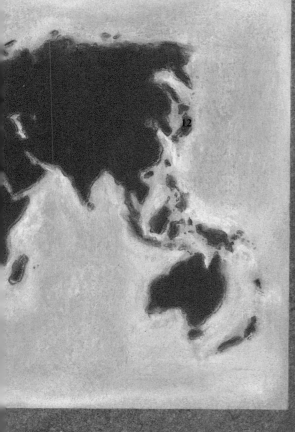

A special thanks to the following: students at Pratt and Duckrey Schools in Philadelphia, Pennsylvania; Winthrop Grade School in Winthrop, Maine; Webster and Lake Street Schools in Auburn, Maine; Agassiz School in Jamacia Plains, Massachusetts; John Marshall Middle School in Indianapolis, Indiana; Lisa Earlbaum; Jay Hoffman; Patricia Stanton; the Moraga Family; Kate McGiff; Steve Saunders; Justine Denison; the Reinsborough Family; James Young; Walter Taranko; Roddy Forsyth; Keven Kelley; Peter Kiang; Joli Green; Lisa Hayden; Joan Benoit Samuelson; Sara Duncan; Karen Richards Toothaker; Bill and Jane Britt; Bob Katz; Ian Foster; Sandy Nevens; Jean and John Sibley; Winnie and Alec McPhedran; Wilasinee Auonkham; Ruth McCaslin; Junko Tomimoto; Andres Oscare; Nicole Bruyere; Richard Parker; Alison Kenway; the Shed-Davis Family; Fiona Knox; Michelle Gifford; Sheila Wilensky-Lanford; Patricia Chaleo; Vivian Wai-Fun Lee; Hildie Lipson; Dara Lay; Barbara Brown; and Gretchen Walsh.

Tilbury House, Publishers
132 Water Street
Gardiner, Maine 04345

Copyright © 1996 by Margy Burns Knight.
Illustrations Copyright © 1996 by Anne Sibley O'Brien

All rights reserved. No part of this publication may be reproduced or transmitted in any form or by any means, electronic or mechanical, including photocopying, recording, or information storage or retrieval systems, without permission in writing from the publisher.

First Edition, June 1996
10 9 8 7 6 5 4 3 2 1

Art direction, design: Susan Sherman, Ars Agassiz, Cambridge, Massachusetts, based on the original design of *Talking Walls* (1992), by Edith Allard, Crummet Mountain, Somerville, Maine.
Editorial: Mark Melnicove, Jennifer Elliott.
Office: Jolene Collins.
Sales and marketing: Michelle Gifford.
Warehouse: William Hoch.
Color separations: Graphic Color, Fairfield, Maine.
Printing and binding: Worzalla, Stevens Point, Wisconsin.

Library of Congress Cataloging-in-Publication Data:

Knight, Margy Burns.
Talking walls : the stories continue / by Margy Burns Knight ; illustrated by Anne Sibley O'Brien.
    p. cm.
Summary: Introduces different cultures around the world by telling the stories of walls, from the Maya murals in Bonampak, Mexico, to dikes in the Netherlands.
ISBN 0-88448-164-5 (he : alk. paper)
    1. Walls—Juvenile literature. 2. Human geography—Juvenile literature. [1. Walls. 2. Human geography.] I. O'Brien, Anne Sibley, ill. II. Title TH2201.K6419 1996
900—dc20   96—15123
                                            CIP
                                            AC

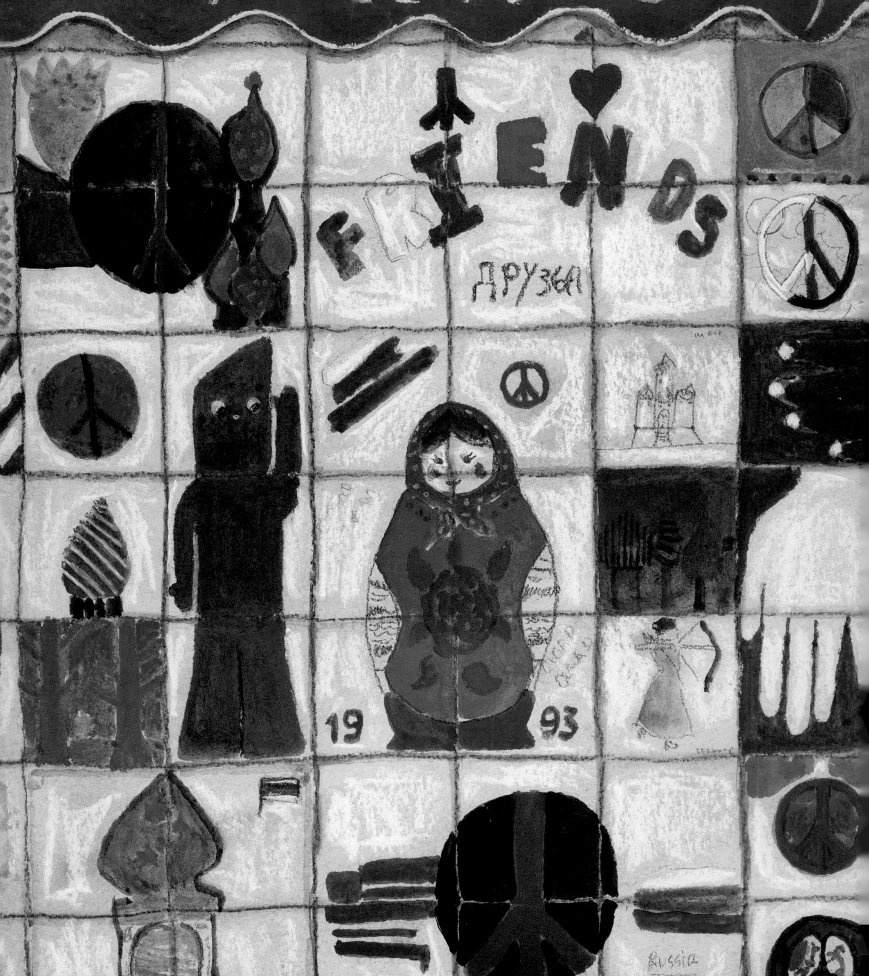